WEIGHT LOSS LIFE

IN TEN EASY STEPS

Todd Singleton, D.C.
Patrick K. Porter, Ph.D.

For information about Club Reduce® Self-Mastery Technology
please visit: **www.Self-MasteryTechnology.com**

Cover Art: Jason Rina
Editor: Heidi Porter

Disclaimer: This book is designed to provide information in regard to the subject matter covered. It is sold with the understanding that the publisher and author are not engaged in rendering psychological advice. This book is not intended to diagnose, treat, cure or prevent any disease. Consult your physician before taking any health supplement. Result may vary by individual. The processes in this book are non-diagnostic and non-psychological. If psychological or other expert assistance is required, the services of a licensed professional should be sought. The purpose of this book is to educate and entertain. The publisher, author, or any dealer or distributor shall not be liable to the purchaser or any other person or entity with respect to any liability, loss, or damage caused or alleged to be caused directly or indirectly by this book. **If you do not wish to be bound by the above, you may return this book for a full refund.**

First Edition: Febuary 2011

ISBN:978-1-4507-5444-6
Library of Congress Control Number: Pending
Printed in the United States of America
10 9 8 7 6 5 4 3

TABLE OF CONTENTS

DEDICATION

This book is dedicated to the truth seeker. The person who isn't satisfied with just surviving but wants to thrive with abundant health, energy and wellbeing.

ACKNOWLEDGEMENT

When I started working with Dr. Singleton and the Club Reduce doctors to bring the Self-Mastery Technology (SMT) component to their already successful weight loss and wellness programs, I realized that I had tapped into a wellspring of knowledge on nutrition and health that needed to be shared with the millions of Americans fighting the battle of the bulge. This book is a collaboration of many, and is meant to touch the lives of as many individuals as possible.

I would like to thank everyone who put their hearts and souls into this project, starting with Dr. Todd Singleton, DC and his wife Nancy, who is not only the brains behind the formation of the Club Reduce system, but also a visionary for the Chiropractic field and its role in the changing world of wellness.

Thanks also go out to Kristi Frank who has been a guiding light in the business community and kindly wrote the foreward to this book.

In my journey of writing books over the last 25 years, I have come to rely on the talents of my family. Thankfully, I have a large family, which means I have plenty of help. I would like to acknowledge my wife, Cynthia, for her help and encouragement in putting the text together and sharing her special gift as a writer. Thanks to my sister-in law, Heidi Porter, for accepting the challenge editing.

Thanks, too, to Jason Rina, for sharing his exceptional artistic talent in the design of this book cover.

FOREWORD

I've been fortunate to have some truly amazing business experiences in my life so far.

Being on the first season of Donald Trump's "The Apprentice" was one of those fantastic experiences.

Because of that exposure, even more business opportunities have opened up for me. That has caused my life and schedule to become very demanding.

On top of a demanding business schedule, I'm also busy raising my son with my husband.

One of the reasons I am able to keep up with such a challenging schedule is that my health has always been a priority to me.

Several years ago, my husband and I decided to leave the fast paced life of LA for a more family friendly environment in the pristine mountains of Park City, Utah. Although I am well versed on principles of healthy living, I'm wise enough to know that it's a good idea to have a doctor on my side who is looking out for my best interest. After my move to Park City, I needed to find a new doctor in the area, who could help me when I needed it.

I had heard about Dr. Todd Singleton, D.C. who has helped thousands of patients, lectures nationwide and teaches other doctors his energy and health promoting systems. At the time I went to see Dr. Singleton, I had a particularly stressful and demanding schedule; and that was taking its toll on my body.

As a wife, mother and entrepreneur I found myself taking care of everyone and ignoring some of the things I needed.

Utilizing the principles taught in his clinic, Club Reduce®, Dr. Singleton was able to look at what was going on with me and help get me right back into balance and living the way that I know is best.

If you are ready to turn your life around and take control, I'd admonish you to find a Club Reduce® doctor in your area who can help you to look your best and achieve the dreams and goals you have for yourself!

Kristi Frank

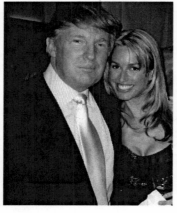 Kristi Frank from Season #1 of NBC's 'The Apprentice,' is well known for helping women entrepreneurs start and grow their online businesses. Kristi has been featured on 'Oprah,' 'MSNBC,' 'The Today Show' and 'The View.' She is currently following her entrepreneurial spirit in many business endeavors including promoting and hosting online success shows for entrepreneurs.

Introduction
by Dr. Todd G. Singleton

I asked my wife, Nancy, to marry me on our third date. We'd only been seeing each other about a week, yet I knew she was the only woman for me.

I know such impulsiveness may seem crazy to some people, but in our case, it all worked out. My wife and I have been happily married for twenty-eight years and have four wonderful children.

Because ours was such a whirlwind romance, most life choices were never discussed before our wedding, including my profession. We were young and in love, and we didn't focus much on the future. It was all about how blissfully happy we were. One day Nancy asked me nonchalantly, "What are your career goals?"

"Don't worry, whatever I do, I'll be the best at it," I replied.

That was all she needed to hear.

At the time, I was just about to start school. I was working in construction, so I had plans to study in that field. Two weeks into our marriage, the contractor I was working for went out of business. I was left without work and no idea what to do next. I spent the day worrying about how I would break the news to my new wife.

Later that night, I sat down with Nancy and told her the truth.

She touched my face and smiled. "I don't care where you work or what you do," she said. "I just won't be married to someone who doesn't absolutely love what they do." She looked me square in the eye. "So, what's your passion? What do you want to be when you grow up?"

The answer was on the tip of my tongue, yet I hesitated. To accomplish that dream would take years of schooling and cost thousands of dollars. We'd have to take out student loans. I would have to spend hours studying every day. I shook my head.

"Tell me," she said.

"I want to be a chiropractor." It was all I ever wanted to be, but what would Nancy think of the idea?

"Then let's do it," she said with a smile.

That night we made up our minds to reach for my dream, and neither of us ever looked back or regretted it. I've been able to change countless lives by helping people gain freedom from their pain. The rewards in our lives are beyond measure.

About six years ago, after I had been practicing for fifteen years, Nancy, asked me the same question that she had asked me years ago: "What is your passion?"

While I love being a chiropractor and enjoy the satisfaction in relieving my patients' pain, what I'd become more passionate about was seeing sick, exhausted, unhappy patients regain their health, vibrancy and zest for life. I'm not talking about simply eliminating pain; I'm talking about people going from feeling really sick to feeling radiant.

There's no greater high than watching patients' lives change. I've seen women too sick to get pregnant regain their health and finally conceive. I've seen diabetics get off their insulin. I've seen dark circles vanish and faces brighten as patients who'd been exhausted from chronic insomnia finally sleep. I've had patients who'd previously had so little energy they could barely make it to my office transformed into healthy, energetic people with fulfilling lives.

I've seen chronic skin problems clear up, digestive problems disappear, people with low libido get their drive back, children labeled ADHD calm down and cope well in school, and people who had no hope for a healthy life regain their health and vitality.

So when my wife asked me, "What is your passion?"

My reply was, "I am passionate about changing peoples' lives. I want to focus on getting people healthy. I want to open up a wellness clinic."

My wife, who loves business and is very good at it, had an odd look on her face. "Fine," she said, "but more people care about losing weight than getting healthy. Why don't you open up a clinic that helps people lose weight and they'll get healthy at the same time?"

Of course! Nearly all my patients who got healthy also lost weight and all my patients who lost weight got healthier. Nancy's suggestion made perfect sense!

Now, thousands of healthier, happier and slimmer patients later, I'm very grateful for that advice.

I've seen patients lose a hundred pounds and more. But what's interesting is how they invariably end up being more excited about how great they feel, rather than how great they look. It was their weight problem that brought them in, and they are thrilled with their new bodies, but they are even more grateful for their improved health overall.

By following the Club Reduce® program, that's what will happen with you, too.

Right now, you are motivated by losing weight. And using this system, you will lose weight. If you're like most of my patients, though, you will be even more thrilled by how great you feel.

I have personally helped thousands of patients go through this program, but everywhere I turned I saw more people who needed my help. That's when I decided to start teaching this system to doctors across the country. Today I am personally acquainted with hundreds of doctors who are also helping thousands of patients change their lives using the Club Reduce® principles.

We have a message and we have a mission. We are changing this country one life at a time. Now it's your turn to change.

Sure, you are going to look great. That's what drove you to us. You want to lose weight; you want to fit into that special dress or look great for your upcoming reunion.

Yep, that will happen. But it's not the reason we do this.

This is about you getting healthy. This is about your life changing. This is about you having all the energy you need to fulfill your life's purpose.

It's interesting that we are almost brainwashed to believe it doesn't matter what we put into our bodies.

When I was in kindergarten, my class took a field trip to the zoo. We were encouraged to feed the elephants, birds and monkeys and we'd give them morsels of our soft white bread or potato chips.

Well guess what happened?

Those poor zoo animals started getting sick. They came down with stomach problems, tumors and yes, even cancer. Signs at the zoo now warn, "Don't feed the animals!" We wouldn't dream of giving animals such unhealthy food. It would kill them; it would be animal cruelty. Yet we still feed that spongy white bread and those fat-laden potato chips to our kindergarteners and we continue to eat that junk ourselves.

And then we wonder why we are sick, tired, lethargic, moody, depressed and fat!

Listen, I know this is a tough subject. Most of us have strong emotional ties to food. When you were a baby and you cried, your mother fed you. It was the beginning of an emotional attachment to food that spans a lifetime. Take away someone's food, and you take away his or her comfort.

We know you think losing weight is hard. We know that you're reading this book because all other methods have failed you.

But don't worry. We've discovered the secrets to success. The tools we have for you will help you succeed just like the thousands of people who have gone ahead of you.

You can lose weight, but it's hard to figure it all out on your own, especially when you are so emotionally attached to food.

But that's why we're here. Together we are going to teach you just what you need to know. We'll teach you, "Weight Loss for Life in 10 Easy Steps."

Let's get started!

CHAPTER

O N E

ACCOUNTABILITY

Accountability!

If You Could Lose Weight On Your Own, You Wouldn't Be Reading this Book!

Years ago, when I first opened up my weight-loss clinic, I thought I had all the answers; I'd just tell my patients what they should eat, the supplements they should take, the amount of sleep to get, the amount of water to drink, the type of exercise to do, and they'd go home and do it.

I believed that after their first office visit they would simply follow my advice, lose weight and get healthy. And why wouldn't they? I was the doctor, after all, and shouldn't patients do what their doctor recommends?

Well, it wasn't that simple. What I hadn't taken into account was that people who are overweight eat for reasons other than hunger. I had also had not recognized that people who are overweight have developed ingrained eating habits that must be changed before they can succeed.

The good news is, those other reasons can be resolved and even deep-rooted habits can be changed. I've seen people do it.

Doctors from across the country who come to learn the Club Reduce® system, often ask me, "What's your secret...why are your patients doing so well?"

I tell them that one of the biggest differences between Club Reduce and a diet or commercial weight loss program is that we provide accountability for our patients.

By adding a weekly accountability meeting to my program, my patients did much better. I don't let patients to go more than a few days without some type of contact from my office. I typically like them to come in once a week and then to get a call from us once a week between office visits. Habit changes are much easier when people are held accountable.

Why is accountability so magical?

Think about it. Since we were children, we performed better when we were held accountable. You brushed your teeth because you knew that before you went to bed your mom would ask you, "Did you brush your teeth?" But if mom were away, or if you were at a sleepover or at camp, the teeth definitely did not get brushed.

Think back to school. You studied for tests because of the accountability factor. You knew someone was going to check up on your knowledge of the subject and you would be graded based on that accountability. Did you ever do extra reading in your history book or extra math problems that weren't assigned? Probably not—if there was no accountability attached. We are motivated to do those things for which we know we will be held accountable. Even as adults, we need that accountability.

My wife gives a great example of the benefit of accountability.

The church we attend asks its members to look out for their neighbors. Both men and women are given assignments to help "look out for" at least three neighbors. For example, Nancy has been assigned three women in our neighborhood to "look out for." Each month, she is to call, visit, send a note or just do something nice for them. It's a good system. Everybody looks out for each other. That way, if anyone has a problem, there is always someone they can turn to in the neighborhood.

Nancy believes this is a great idea and she's happy to do it. Who doesn't think helping your neighbor is a good thing? Nobody would argue with that. We all want to be good neighbors and friends.

But as my wife points out, while she is happy to help her neighbors, what works best to ensure she will remember to contact them as assigned is a monthly accountability check—a call she gets at the end of each month from someone else who was given the task of checking up on her to make sure she followed through with her commitment.

Aren't we adults? Shouldn't we just follow through on what we volunteered to do? Yes, but as they say, "The road to hell is paved with good intentions." How many good things do we intend to do, but forget to do because we are too busy or distracted?

In this case, someone calls Nancy to get an accounting of what happened. While she has good intentions to visit or send a note to the three women she is assigned, she follows through because she has to answer to someone else about her assignment. So while she wants to do the right thing, she is driven to do it because she would be embarrassed to get the monthly phone call and say, "No, I dropped the ball, I didn't contact my assigned neighbor."

Accountability works!

When I was a young married student, we lived in apartments. My wife made friends with a young woman in one of the apartments close to ours. The pair decided they would walk together every morning at 5:00 a.m. Her friend would knock on our door at 5:00 and off they'd go.

But if her friend was ever out of town, my wife didn't go. She could have gone walking alone. She knew she should exercise, but it was the accountability of her friend that ensured she went.

Again, accountability works. It's just that plain and simple.

Not only do we follow through when someone checks up on us, we actually do better. This phenomenon was shown to be true by studies in the early 20th Century that brought about the phrase the "Hawthorne Effect."

The experiment took place from 1924 to 1932 at Hawthorne Works, a Western Electric factory outside Chicago. Researchers increased and decreased certain variables in the workers' environment and then measured productivity levels. The variable that produced the most productivity gain was the motivational effect of the interest being shown in them. Workers' productivity improved simply because they were being monitored.

Ah, hah!

No wonder accountability is so important. Showing interest in someone on a weight-loss program actually helps that person stick with the success system and get better results.

Sounds easy, and it is. You are overweight because you have developed lifestyle habits that caused you to gain weight. It is definitely possible to change a habit, but often difficult when you attempt this on your own. When you have someone to whom you are accountable, you are more likely to follow through.

Do you ever remember wanting to do something, but being unsure as to whether or not you could do it? For example, do you remember the first time you jumped off a diving board into a swimming pool? Odds are you were afraid, but a friend, sibling or parent was probably standing by saying, "Come on you can do it...of course you can do it....just do it...jump!"

Eventually the trust someone else had in you was enough motivation to get you to actually jump into the water, even though you were afraid.

The same thing is true with weight-loss.

More than likely this is not the first place you've looked for a solution to your weight problem. You have probably tried many diets and gimmicks and failed.

So now, here you are, reading this book thinking: I don't know if I can do this. I've tried so many times and nothing's worked. How do I know this will work? How do I know if this program is right for me?

You are asking yourself all of these questions, and the fact is, you want this to work, but you have doubts...doubts in yourself and doubts that this program will be any different or better.

The Club Reduce program is different because it teaches you how to make lifestyle changes that will lead to weight-loss and pristine health! And, lucky for you, we are here to be your accountability partner.

We've helped thousands and thousands of patients lose their weight. We know this program works, so we are here to say, "You can do it, of course you can...others have...now it's your turn...come on, do it!"

This is one of those times when you simply need someone to keep you accountable and say, "You can do it!" (Because you can, we know it, and we'll help you until you know it!)

Women especially are guilty of taking care of everyone but themselves. They are used to doing for their children and sacrificing. Women are amazing! But sometimes, because their nature is that of nurturer, they are used to putting others' needs first. Unfortunately, this often translates into not taking care of themselves.

Women do well with an accountability partner who can say, "Do this. You need to do it for yourself. You can stick with this. It's your turn!" Sometimes the little extra push from an accountability partner will be the difference in success or failure!

We will have you keep an accountability journal of everything you are assigned to do to stick with the program every day. Through the years, we have found that when a patient is doing everything they can, they are excited to bring their accountability journal into the office so we can see what they are doing.

One afternoon we were having a staff meeting and all patients were on their way out of our office. One gentleman in his 60's lingered. He said, "Nobody looked at my journal."

That was very revealing. He wanted us to see his progress. He wanted a gold star for his hard work. It reminded me of a little child who wanted his mother to look at his beautiful drawing. We all want recognition when we are doing something well.

If someone shows up at our office and doesn't have their accountability journal, we know they are really saying, "I didn't do well, so I don't want you to see what I've done." We'll say, "Go home and get it. We want to see it."

Hey, this is a learning process. By seeing what you are doing, we are better able to offer suggestions.
Once someone knows they are going to be held accountable, they'll stick with it and succeed.

There are many other steps in the process that are very important, but accountability is one of the most important.

Again, if you could have done this on your own, you wouldn't be reading this book.

Now together, as your accountability partner, we will help you, and you will succeed!

CHAPTER
TWO

Food and Digestion

DIET

Most Americans are eating an imbalanced diet. What is advertised as a balanced diet and what the laws of nature define as a balanced diet are total opposites. In truth, most Americans consume a diet of devitalized, over processed, over cooked, over refined, and filled with chemicals. These are consumed with toxic items such as sugar, salt, chocolate, carbonated drinks, pastries, pies, coffee, tobacco and alcohol. A combination of these things combined with polluted air and other negative environmental factors bring about a general deterioration of health, biochemical imbalance, and systemic disturbances leading to metabolic disorders and pathological changes to the tissues and joints of the body as well as body obesity.

Dr. Weston A. Price performed extensive studies of health and dietary habits of every race of people throughout the world. He came to the conclusion that the condition of their health is directly related to the foods they eat. In his book, Nutrition and Physical Degeneration, he stated that wherever he found strong, healthy, disease free and tooth decay free people he also found that their diets were made up of natural, fresh, pure and unprocessed foods available in their immediate environment. Conversely, wherever he found people subject to the various diseases common to civilized man, including tooth decay, he invariably found that they ate denatured, cooked, processed foods that included white sugar, white bread and canned foods, which had found their way to them from the more affluent civilized countries.

Many people, including health professionals, think that Americans have the safest food in the world. The truth is that Americans are the most overfed and undernourished people on the earth today. The foods we eat can contribute to immune system suppression which can cause everything from arthritis to weight gain. There are very few foods in our supermarkets that do not have sugar, preservatives, artificial colors and artificial sweeteners added. We have processed the goodness out of our foods, increased our fat intake, decreased our dietary fiber, and added harmful ingredients and chemicals to an incredibly high amount of food we eat.

We'll begin by talking about the foods and food additives that are harmful to our bodies, causing all manner of disease and weight gain; and which fail to properly nourish our bodies and keep us healthy. The following sections are an outline of some of the worst enemies to our bodies and to the immune system in the American diet.

SUGAR

When a person eats simple sugars the immune system is compromised. Refined white sugar triggers the release of insulin from the pancreas. With daily consumption of sugar, the blood stream is always laced with insulin, which suppresses the secretion of growth hormone from the pituitary gland. Both insulin and growth hormone are inversely related; insulin is a fat making hormone while growth hormone is a fat burning hormone. Growth hormone is a prime regulator of the immune system. In addition to being an immune system suppressant, sugar also feeds Candida by helping yeast to thrive. The ingestion of as little as 100 grams of refined sugar reduces the ability of the white blood cells to destroy bacteria. There is at least a 50% reduction within two hours of eating sugar. The average American ingests at least 150 grams of sucrose in addition to other refined sugars every day. It is easy to conclude that most Americans have depressed immune systems.

Besides suppressing the immune system, sugar causes other harmful effects in the body. Sugar upsets the mineral balance in the body. Sugar can cause hyperactivity, anxiety, concentration difficulties and crankiness in children. Sugar can produce a significant rise in triglycerides.

Sugar contributes to the reduction of the defense against bacterial infection. Sugar leads to chromium deficiency. Sugar leads to cancer of the breast, ovaries, prostate and rectum. Sugar can increase fasting levels of glucose. Sugar causes copper deficiency. Sugar interferes with the absorption of calcium and magnesium. Sugar raises the level of a neuro-transmitter called serotonin. Sugar can cause hypoglycemia . Sugar can produce an acidic stomach. Sugar can lead to alcoholism. Sugar causes tooth decay. Sugar contributes to obesity. The high intake of sugar increases the risk of Crohn's Disease and ulcerative colitis . Sugar can cause changes frequently found in persons with gastric or duodenal ulcers.

Sugar can cause arthritis. Sugar can cause asthma, Candida Albicans, gallstones, appendicitis, hemorrhoids, periodontal disease , contributes to osteoporosis, causes a decrease in insulin sensitivity, decreased glucose tolerance, decreased growth hormone; can increase cholesterol, increases the systolic blood pressure, can cause drowsiness and decreased activity in children; causes migraine headaches, interferes with the absorption of protein, causes food allergies and also contributes to diabetes; causes toxemia during pregnancy, eczema in children, impairs the structure of DNA, changes the structure of proteins and alters the way they act in the body; can make the structure of collagen in our skin change; causes cataracts; promotes an elevation of low density proteins; causes free radicals in the blood stream; lowers the enzymes' ability to function; can cause loss of tissue elasticity and function; increases the size of the liver by making the cells divide; increase kidney size and produce pathological changes in the kidneys; can overstress or damage the pancreas; increases the body's fluid retention; can compromise the lining of the capillaries; can make the tendons more brittle; can an increase in delta, alpha and theta brain waves; causes depression; increases the risk of gastric cancers and gallbladder cancer, of getting gout; increases bacterial fermentation in the colon; increases the risk of colon cancer in women; causes platelet adhesiveness ; can cause hormonal imbalances. Sugar can also lead to the formation of kidney stones. Is it any wonder we should be concerned about the increasing amounts of this toxic substance we are ingesting?

ARTIFICIAL SWEETENERS

Artificial sweeteners are acidifying. The bad guys include aspartame, nutra sweet, saccharine, sweet n low, sucralose, splenda, sweet and safe, sweet one, and clamates. They all break down into deadly acids in the body. For example, when you ingest aspartame, one of the ingredients, methyl alcohol, converts to formaldehyde, a deadly neuro-toxin, as well as a known carcinogen .

That's not all. From there it turns to formic acid, which is, by the way, the poison fire ants use when they attack. That's just one ingredient of many of the artificial sweeteners. A wide variety of symptoms can be caused by artificial sweeteners, including headaches, migraines, dizziness, vertigo, seizures, depression, fatigue, irritability, increased heart rate, heart palpitations, insomnia, vision problems, hearing loss, ringing the in ears, weight gain, numbness, muscle spasms, joint pain, breathing difficulty, anxiety attacks, slurred speech and a loss of taste.

There are also a lot of artificial sweeteners that are toxic to the body. Aspartame is one of the worst. Far from saving us calories, these artificial chemicals are wreaking havoc in our bodies. In 1994 the US Department of Health and Human Services, DHHS, released a listing of adverse reactions to aspartame reported to the FDA. The most common reactions include abdominal pain, anxiety attacks, arthritis, asthma, bloating, blood sugar control problems, breathing difficulties, burning eyes and throat, irregular urination, chronic fatigue, confusion, depression, dizziness, hair loss, headaches, migraines, heart palpations, hives, high blood pressure, infections, impotency, insomnia, irritability, itching, joint pain, memory loss, hormone imbalance, seizures, muscle spasms, nausea, numbness or tingling of extremities, allergic reactions, panic attacks, tremors, tinnitus , and vertigo; as well as causing weight gain.

The reactions from this one chemical accounted for more than 75% of all adverse reactions reported to the FDA's adverse reaction monitoring system.   Aspartame overuse mimics symptoms and worsens the following diseases: Fibroidmyalgia, arthritis, multiple sclerosis, Parkinson's disease, lupus, diabetes, epilepsy, Alzheimer's, chronic fatigue, Lyme's disease, lypoma , attention deficit disorder and depression.

It often takes at least sixty days without aspartame to see significant improvement, as it is a chemical drug that stays in the body for a very long time without a dramatic cleanse such as detoxification.

Artificial sweeteners can also trigger or worsen arthritis, chronic fatigue, diabetes, Fibroidmyalgia, brain tumors, MS, Parkinson's, Alzheimer's, systemic lupus, mental retardation, birth defects, thyroid disorders, lymphoma and epilepsy. Don't let them enter your body to do their worst. Safer sweeteners to use would be natural plant sources, such as the herb Stevia, Chicory (which you can find in your natural food store), or the Solutions4 Simply Sweet.

MSG-Monosodium Glutamate

MSG is also known as gelatin, hydrolyzed vegetable protein, textured protein and yeast extracts. Sodium salt of the amino acid glutamic acid or glutamate, MSG, is an additive used to enhance the flavor of foods. Basically, it makes cheap food taste great. It does not have a flavor of its own but it stimulates glutamate receptors on the tongue to enhance the tastes of foods.

The side effects of MSG include headaches, weakness, muscle aches, numbness, tingling, flushing and allergies. Fibroidmyalgia, candida and all other autoimmune disorders respond to a diet of MSG and aspartame elimination by a significant relation of the symptoms of the syndrome.

CAFFEINE

One of the worst offenders in the modern American diet is caffeine. Found in sodas, drugs and coffee, the diuretic properties of caffeine rob the body of potassium and other important minerals and cleansing fluids. In addition, while robbing our bodies of necessary liquids as a diuretic, we often drink even less water (that we desperately need) because we're no longer thirsty after consuming a soda or cup of coffee. This further dehydrates the system.

Remember the days when we used to talk about our problems over a cup of coffee? Now, coffee is the problem. Rather than getting the edge, we have found that coffee makes us edgy. Some people drink three cups of coffee, a few sodas and take a couple of Excedrin all in the course of a morning. That accounts to over 500 milligrams of caffeine. Is it any wonder that tranquilizers are one of the most prevalent drugs prescribed in America? In fact, one in seven adult Americans takes some sort of tranquilizer to calm their nerves. Taking stimulants along with tranquilizers is like driving with your foot on the gas and the brake at the same time. It's all too easy for doctors to misdiagnose a case of excessive caffeine consumption as anxiety neurosis caused by emotional factors.

Coffee is the number one drink in America, with six out of ten adults drinking it every day. Caffeine is one of the most widely used drugs in America and it has no nutritional value. With this wonder drug people think they can get the jump on their fellow man. Teenagers love soda and account for 25% of the total caffeine consumption, which is a number that is continuing to climb. It is estimated that 30% of Americans take between 500 to 600 milligrams of caffeine per day and 10% use more than 1000 milligrams per day. The average person, including children, consumes 200 milligrams per day. One cup of coffee contains 100-150 milligrams and one to two cups exceed the level at which your brain can be adversely affected; not to mention the new high-caffeine soft drinks that they have touted as "energy drinks". Habituation is caffeine's secret of success. Caffeine enters all the organs and tissues of the body within a few minutes of ingestion. 90% is metabolized and only 10% is excreted, unchanged, in urine.

You may be thinking since everyone drinks coffee, tea and Coke, that it can't be that bad. Well, it's time to understand some of the side effects of caffeine; if you are having any of these symptoms we're about to describe, you may be smart to discontinue consuming anything with caffeine. Caffeine may be subtle and obscured by the multi factored natures of many chronic disease states. For a better understanding, we have categorized how caffeine affects all the systems of the body.

Caffeine has serious effects on the nervous system. In children it may cause damage to the brain and central nervous system development. A survey revealed that even pregnant women consumed an average of 193 milligrams of caffeine per day. Over 400,000 pregnant women (which is 13% of pregnant women) drink five or more cups of coffee per day, causing thousands of birth defects.

Caffeine is a powerful central nervous system stimulant. Large doses may impair motor function where delicate coordination is required. It increases reaction to sensory stimuli but the post stimulation produces a let-down effect which results in fatigue, lethargy and depression. High doses can produce symptoms indistinguishable from anxiety neurosis.

Caffeine can cause nervousness, irritability, jitteriness, muscle tension and trembling. It can cause headaches, shaky hands and even hallucinations. Caffeine is the principle cause of restless leg syndrome, which results in insomnia and an uncomfortable feeling caused by involuntary movement of the legs. Children have increased hyperactivity and insomnia from Cocoa drinks and sodas. Many parents can't figure out why their kids are out of control and why the kids have trouble settling down to sleep at night. Many times, the reason is due to the amount of caffeine they consume.

Caffeine has significant effects on muscle contractions, relaxing smooth muscle and increasing the contraction of skeletal muscles. Caffeine may mask mental and physical fatigue. This may be dangerous if used while driving. It is not a substitute for normal rest or sleep. Caffeine may interact with other drugs; and it decreases drug induced sleeping time.

Caffeine is habit-forming and addictive. Thiamine and Vitamin B-1 is destroyed by both coffee and teas. Any heavy coffee drinker is likely to be deficient in B-1, which is crucial for mental health and tranquility. It is called the morale vitamin. Lack of Thiamine causes nervous exhaustion and fatigue, loss of appetite, loss of memory, depression, constipation, inability to concentrate, feelings of inadequacy, lethargy and intense drowsiness.

Through its actions, caffeine can trigger psychosis on a set of chemicals in the brain called neurotransmitters. Neurotransmitters convey information across microscopic gaps called synapses between nerve cells in the brain. Caffeine causes significant changes in these different transmitter systems. Caffeine, even in moderate doses, is a threat to your mental health. All mental and physical stimulation ceases if you consume more than two cups at a time. After two cups coffee caffeine acts to slow your reaction time and impair your thinking. Caffeine could well be one of the most frequent causes of chronic recurrent headaches. Ten grams, which is found in only forty cups of coffee, may cause grand mal seizures, respiratory failure and death.

Caffeine's affect on the heart and circulatory systems increases the free fatty acids causing an increase in blood fats and cholesterol associated with heart attacks and other cardiovascular disease. Caffeine can cause heart palpitations and light headedness. It can cause flushing as it dilates the blood vessels. Caffeine can case tachycardia , rapid heart rate, arrhythmias , and irregular heart beat as caffeine stimulates the cardiac muscle.

Caffeine consumption can cause coronary disease, heart disease and high blood pressure. There is an increase of myocardial infarction (lack of blood supply to the heart) among coffee drinkers. There is a 60% increase in heart attacks associated with the consumption of one to five cups per day and 120% increase with more than five cups per day. Yet some coronary care units still serve coffee, tea and cola drinks. Heart specialists have recognized caffeine as a mild poison.

Caffeine's effect on the gastrointestinal system increases the amount of hydrochloric acid in the stomach causing hyper acidity. This accounts for the burning sensation reported by ulcer patients. There is a 72% greater chance of developing ulcers in coffee drinkers compared to non drinkers. Caffeine aggravates the symptoms of peptic ulcers . Coffee drinkers are twice as likely to develop pancreatic cancer than non users. Coffee could cause more than half of the cancers of the pancreas in the US according to Harvard researchers. This deadly form of cancer takes the lives of 20,000 Americans annually, with less than a 1% survival rate in the past five years. One to two cups per day doubles the risk. Three or more triple the risk. Caffeine intake has also been linked to prostate cancer.

Caffeine affects how your body absorbs iron, which can lead to anemia. Strong coffee takes twice as much iron from being absorbed; using cream in your coffee worsens this effect. Caffeine accumulates in the body in liver disease. Caffeine is a possible stimulating factor in the cancer of the stomach. It stimulates the secretion of the small intestines and stimulates water secretion and can cause nausea and loose stools. It can cause hypoglycemia response in the presence of glucose and it elevates blood glucose.

Caffeine alters the metabolic status of human beings and can increase your metabolic rate 10-25% with 500 milligrams of caffeine; this is to metabolize the caffeine out of your body. Caffeine is absorbed into your bloodstream and even passing the blood-brain barrier. The half life of caffeine in the human body is between 3 to 7 hours. Females metabolize caffeine 20-30% more quickly than males. However, it will take women on "the pill" twice as long to metabolize caffeine as women who are ovulating. When we say caffeine increases your metabolism, this does not mean that it burns fat, but requires increased energy to burn up that toxin from your body. Ever wonder why you need another caffeine boost later?

Caffeine can also affect the kidney, bladder and prostate. A study at Harvard University showed a correlation between caffeine and cancer of the bladder. Cola drinkers have a significant increase in bladder cancer. A drastic example of the devastating effects of caffeine on the human body was fluid retention, which persisted ten years, caused by ingestion of eighteen cups of coffee a day by a patient who complained of being a nervous wreck. All symptoms disappeared when she quit coffee.

FDA scientists are advising pregnant women to avoid caffeine-containing foods and drugs. They are considering putting a warning on coffee to pregnant woman due to the risk of fetal malformations. Coffee crosses the placenta to the baby and is passed into the breast milk. Birth defects may include cleft palate, digit defects, joint defects, absence of jaw, unusual smallness of lower jaw, blood tumors, club feet and delayed skeletal development. In England, ectrodactyly, a congenital absence of all or part of the fingers or toes, has been connected to heavy coffee consumption during pregnancy. In large doses, it has been shown to be a mutagen in animals, plants and bacteria. Caffeine may also cause miscarriages.

How do you know if you're addicted to caffeine? A simple test would be to stop using it for two or three days. If you have a caffeine addiction you will likely experience the following symptoms: headaches starting about eighteen hours after your last consumption; drowsiness and almost overwhelming malaise; lethargy; runny nose and nausea; a cotton feeling in the mouth; nervousness and irritability; trembling with a chill; insomnia; depression; and an inability to work effectively. These withdrawal symptoms can last up to two weeks or more depending on how much you have consumed and your age.

What about caffeine free products? Aren't they a better alternative? A chemical used in making decaffeinated coffee, trichloroethylene (TCE), has been known to cause liver cancer, making caffeine free products an unsafe alternative to caffeinated ones. The National Cancer Institute also warns against using three possible substitutes to TCE. Replacing a chemical with a carcinogenic risk with another chemical of unknown risk may result in a more hazardous alternative. In other words, all the side effects of the chemicals used in decaffeinated coffee are still unknown.

Caffeine free soft drinks and sugar free soft drinks still have substitutes and chemicals. It's best to try to develop a taste for healthy beverages, primarily water. Water is the fluid your body uses to trigger every chemical reaction and enzyme activity in the body. If you don't think a few chemicals in the beverages you consume make any difference in how you feel, try putting one percent water in your gas tank and see how well your car runs. The bottom line is that health is a choice, your choice.

There are alternatives to chemically enhanced and caffeinated beverages. The obvious first choice is fresh spring water. Everyone should drink half their body weight in ounces of water every single day. After strenuous exercise on a hot day, nothing quenches your thirst like water. The juice of fresh lemons in a glass of hot water is also a good way to start the day and is effective in aiding weight loss.

To conquer caffeine addiction, try these tips to lower or avoid intake. Question the impulse. Are you thirsty? Drink water. Do you need to wake up? Breathe deeply, take a brisk walk, do some quick calisthenics. Do you need to feel better? Regular exercise produces more of the natural brain chemicals that improve mood. Are you chronically sleepy or tired? Get more sleep.

One of the things I recommend in my office is the Solutions4 Nutritional shake that comes in chocolate , strawberry, vanilla and orange crème. This is a good caffeine, coffee or soda alternative. Most of my patients are able to get off the caffeine within one to two days by replacing the coffee and soft drinks with a healthy meal replacement alternative that has amino acids, minerals, vitamins and healthy lactose free protein.

HYDROGENATED VEGETABLE OILS

An ingredient in almost all processed foods, baby formulas, non dairy creamers, and dressings is hydrogenated oil. These artificial fats rapidly oxidize in the human system, releasing a deadly barrage of free radicals which can destroy cells and cause genetic damage. They impair the immune system of white blood cells and have been continuously linked to increased risks of cancer.

Fried foods are heavily saturated with fats that are particularly responsible for high blood pressure and heart disease. They can shut down the body's immune mechanism and bring on cancer-causing free radicals as well.

MALNUTRITION

Contrary to common belief, malnutrition is a primary cause of immune deficiency throughout the world; not only in third world countries. Our primary sources of foods in America are fast food restaurants and prepared or packaged foods. Our stomachs feel full, but vitamins and nutrients are extremely minimal. The most glaring deficiencies in modern diets are essential amino acids and essential fatty acids; both of which are required in the production of immune factors such as white blood cells and antibodies.

The thymus gland and the lymph tissue, for example, immediately begin to shrink and atrophy when these nutrients are absent from the diet. An analysis of the US Department of Agriculture's food consumption survey indicates that not a single one of the 20,000 people studied achieved an intake of 100% of the recommended daily allowance, the RDA, of all ten nutrients analyzed.

In other words, no one was getting adequate nutrition from the foods they ate. The lack of single servings each day of fruits and vegetables can add up to a great deficiency over a period of time. Live and unprocessed foods, along with adequate nutrition, are absolutely essential to a life of good health and continual weight loss.

LOW WATER INTAKE

It is essential to consume at least one half of your body weight in ounces of water each day. Water is critical to keep our bodies and our immune systems functioning as they should. Water hydrates and cleanses the cells, while lubricating and flushing out the system. Without proper water intake, waste products build up in the body and impede microcirculation to the skin and decrease the amount of nutrients carried to the cells and organs of the body. Nothing else can take the place of water--not juice, not soda, not alcoholic beverages, coffees, teas or other beverages.

FAD DIETS

One of the most dangerous fad diets today is the no fat obsession. Fats play a crucial role in our bodies and getting none at all opens our bodies up to natural deficiencies and the degeneration that comes with it. The key is to get healthy fats, not the artery clogging, zero nutrient varieties most Americans eat, which are primarily saturated fats and hydrogenated oils. Liquid oils chemically alter into solids. Approximately 20% of your calories should come from healthy fats. What your body needs are essential fatty acids. EFAs are vital to good health. They are the building blocks of the fats that strengthen cell walls. Polyunsaturated fats such as flax, borage, evening primrose oil, grape seed and hemp oils help construct cell membranes, produce hormones and bind and eliminate acids. Most oils contain monounsaturated and polyunsaturated fats, those that are predominantly monounsaturated such as olive oil as well as raw nuts and avocados are also beneficial. They are used for cellular energy, meaning that our body runs on those instead of sugar.

EFAs strengthen immune cells, lubricate joints, insulate the body against heat loss, provide energy and are used to make hormones such as prostoglandulins, which protect against heart disease, stroke, high blood pressure, arteriosclerosis, and blood clots. They are necessary for energy metabolism and immune system health. EFAs can also help relieve arthritis, asthma, PMS, allergies, skin conditions and some behavioral disorders, and also improves brain function.

Nuts, seeds and avocado are excellent sources of healthy fats, including the omega 3s and omega 6s.

REFINED AND PROCESSED FOODS

You've got to skip the junk food. Yes, that means chips, cookies, donuts, and just about anything you get at a fast food restaurant. It also includes many foods you may not have been concerned about before, such as a low calorie frozen dinner, the frozen burrito or the can of soup. All of these things are refined and processed to within an inch of their lives and whatever nutrients they may have had to begin with are trashed in the process; even the so-called enriched products.

On top of that, they are loaded with sugar, salt, artificial color and flavor, additives and preservatives, and butter, margarine or hydrogenated or partially hydrogenated hardened vegetable oil. They are also deficient in fiber. They are, of course, acidifying.

DAIRY PRODUCTS

Like most animal foods, dairy products contain hormone and pesticide residues, microforms , mycotoxins , and saturated fats. Layer on top of that the milk's sugar and lactose, which break down like any sugar and feeds harmful microforms.

Dairy cows feed on stored grains laced with hormones and antibiotics made with fungi which are then concentrated in milk. Also, cheese and yogurt are made by fermentation. Dairy is the leader of all foods in forming sticky mucus. Dairy is acid forming. It can create inflammation in the body which can cause pain. It can increase cancer risks, including ovarian and endometrial. Furthermore, pasteurization destroys the beneficial enzymes milk starts out with. Pasteurization doesn't even actually work. Pasteurized milk left out will rot and stink, whereas raw milk curdles naturally and is still edible.

You can see why all dairy products should be eliminated from your diet. Try soy, almond or rice milk as alternatives. Use unsweetened soy milk to avoid the ones that are filled with added sugar.

If you must have milk, use unprocessed goat's milk from goats that feed on organically grown grass. It contains the antifungal caprylic acid . No matter how many times you were told by teachers and parents to drink your milk, and cute milk mustache ads notwithstanding, the idea that dairy products are healthy is pure hype; a cultural myth.

Even if cows lived in some kind of bovine utopia and produced perfect milk, let's face it. It simply isn't human food. It is designed for baby cows whose requirements are far different from those of humans. Milk is full of components of no use to humans and they must either be converted for use, wasting our body's resources in the process, or eliminated as toxins. No other animal species consumes milk beyond infancy, and certainly not from a species outside their own. Milk is designed for growing babies and not for adults.

Milk is only the beginning of the problem. Consider that it takes ten pounds of milk to make one pound of hard cheese; twelve pounds to make one pound of ice cream; and over twenty one pounds to make one pound of butter. Remember that it takes twenty parts alkalinity to neutralize one part of acidity, just imagine what it takes to counter the effects of so concentrated sources of acid. If it would take twenty cups of something alkaline to neutralize one cup of milk, you would need twelve times as much, (240 cups or 15 gallons) to neutralize a cup of ice cream.

No wonder so many people do so poorly on dairy foods. No

wonder so many people suffer with osteoporosis, while still ingesting so much dairy. No wonder so many people have allergic reactions to dairy or are lactose intolerant. No wonder people gain weight quickly on dairy foods and lose it so quickly when they go off these very concentrated foods. They are just too concentrated and are ultra acidic in the bloodstream.

It is true that Calcium is vital for many functions in the body, but the current rage for getting huge doses of minerals through large quantities of dairy products daily is based on faulty understanding of how the body uses it. Many people worry totally unnecessarily that if milk products are eliminated their diet will leave them deficient in calcium. The fact is that all leafy green vegetables and grasses are inherently high in calcium, as well as iron, magnesium, vitamin C and many of the B vitamins; as are celery, cauliflower, okra, onions, green beans, avocado, black beans, garbanzo beans, chick peas, tofu, almonds, hazelnuts and sesame seeds.

It is important to evaluate how much calcium you really need to keep your bones and body healthy. To do so you must understand that one of the things calcium does in the body is neutralize the acid created by eating animal products. When you eat these acidic foods the body tries to return to its alkaline state the only way it can, by withdrawing calcium from your bones. Your kidneys also rob your bones in order to eliminate the excess nitrogen found in animal protein.

The current recommendations for calcium are 1000 milligrams a day and more; assume an average American diet that consists of 1.5 to 4 times as much protein as necessary, creating an unnatural demand for calcium. Many experts blame the seeming epidemic of bone weakening disease osteoporosis on the protein overdose. It isn't really a lack of calcium at all. Rather it is a calcium robbing problem, not a calcium deficiency problem.

We need to stop worrying about not getting enough calcium and pay attention to not getting too much protein. In the meantime we're all living the irony that getting plenty of calcium rich dairy products can actually leave us with a negative balance but the time all that protein is buffered.

SALT

The negative effects of salt are well known and yet the typical American diet is loaded with it, starting with a salt shaker on probably every dining table in the country. Even if you never use a salt shaker you can easily overdose on salt with processed foods, boxed, bottled, bagged, frozen or canned foods, or restaurant food and junk food; all of which are useless, specifically labeled, and otherwise generally loaded with salt.

Aim to eliminate all added salt from your diet except alkalizing salts like real salt or seasoning salts with vegetables added.

MEAT and EGGS

Animal products and meat such as pork, beef, lamb, chicken, turkey and eggs are filled with hormones, pesticides, steroids, antibiotics, microforms, mycotoxins and the saturated fats that contribute to heart disease, stroke and cancer among many other things . They are highly acidic foods.

These animals feed on stored grain and pass along all the associated problems in their meat. There is a strong correlation between animal protein and several kinds of cancer, particularly breast, ovarian, stomach and colon cancers. Studies show that people who get 70% of their protein from animal products have major health problems compared to those who get just 5% of their protein that way; seventeen times the death rate from heart disease, for example, and five times the likelihood of dying from breast cancer for women.

The consumption of eggs alone is associated with increased risks of colon cancer. Eggs from grain fed chickens have been documented to contain mycotoxins. Dr. Robert O. Young, PhD., observed that fifteen minutes after eating an egg people would begin to show bacteria or an increase in bacteria in their blood. Dairy products were also incriminated in the same study with the highest association being with cheese.

An Australian study also turned up a direct association of egg consumption and colon cancer, as well as links with the intake of red meat, liver, dairy foods and poultry. Researchers studying the effects of a western style diet in Japanese women found that it was linked to a higher risk of breast cancer because of the much larger amounts of meat included. Scientists started down this track after noting that breast cancer was rare in Japanese women before WWII.

Another study linked poultry, ham, salami, bacon and sausage to an increased risk of thyroid cancer as well as cheese, butter and oils other than olive oil. Olive oil is generally free of mycotoxins. Yet another study supported the fact that this type of dietary fat consumed influences the occurrence of endometrial, ovarian and stomach cancers with animal derived fats contributing to an increased risk. People in the study who developed cancer ate more bacon and ham, used more butter in cooking and drank more whole milk.

A Swedish study found a number of dietary factors to be associated with pancreatic cancer including higher consumption of fried and grilled meat. Processed meats and cheeses are even worse, thanks to their nitrosamines , and are a risk factor for brain and spinal cord tumors. Besides, animal foods are simply dead; dead in every aspect, including lack of enzymes. Vegetable foods alive with enzymes, energy and phytonutrients are far superior in every way.

All meats properly aged for human consumption are, by definition, partly fermented and thus permeated with microforms and their toxins. It is yeast, after all, that causes the aging. And the final taste and texture is determined by the nature of the microbial aging process.

Most mycotoxins are heat tolerant so cooking doesn't get rid of them, even if it kills off some of their creators. Automatically and physiologically humans are not meant to be carnivorous or omnivorous. The long complicated human digestive track is designed for the slow absorption of complex and stable plant food. Carnivores have short simple bowels to allow for minimal transit time of unstable dead animal food. Their intestine microorganisms are different from humans too.

On the other side of the coin, starch digestion in humans is quite elaborate, whereas carnivores eat little or no starch. If humans were carnivorous we'd be sweating through our tongues instead of our skin. Flesh eaters have teeth and jaws designed for tearing apart freshly killed animals. Only our hand tools allow us to override this obvious natural limitation; not to mention the fact that we get none of the nutrition contained in fur, feathers, organs or bones the way true carnivores do.

Finally, we seldom eat raw flesh. We commonly need to cook it to kill parasites and other harmful microforms and to disguise the corpse that it is; none of which is necessary for real meat eaters. Humans are designed to be vegetarian. Our bodies will never work at their best if we keep forcing them to do something they are not equipped to handle.

We need to evaluate just how much protein we really need. Expert researchers suggest we need only 25 grams, just one ounce a day of protein. The average American who eats meat, dairy, or eggs probably gets 75 to 125 grams a day; three to five times more than we actually need. Dr. Young recommends that our protein intake should comprise roughly 5-7% of our total diet. Our bodies are just 7% total protein, 70% water, 20% fat, 1-2% vitamins and minerals and 0.5 to 1% sugar. Most meats are 20-25% protein, therefore providing more than the human body requires. If you don't eat meat, never fear. Spinach and other greens are higher in amino acids, the building blocks of protein, than steak. Cow's milk too is protein rich. In contrast, a protein source specifically designed for human consumption, breast milk, is only 5% protein. Some sources produce it as low as 1.4 to 2.2 % protein, and that's meant to be the sole source of nutrition for a human who is growing and developing faster than at any other time of life; doubling or tripling body mass in size within the first year of life.

If we really needed sugar concentrated proteins for good growth and health, surely mother's milk would contain a much higher percentage. Dr. Young believes breast milk percentages more accurately reflect the body's actual requirements. Some of the strongest animals in the world, for example, the gorilla and the elephant, eat no meat. They are obviously not hurting for protein. What do they subsist on? Grass and leaves.

STORED GRAINS

Stored grains mean last year's crop. Grains that are stored will usually begin to ferment within 90 days and in short order are full of mycotoxins. They also harbor harmful microforms. So you want to get this year's crop, preferably within three months of being harvested. Eating stored grains is damaging to the body.

A 1991 study found a direct correlation between eating stored grains and esophageal cancer that same year. Researchers identified cooked cereal, a form of stored grain, as a risk factor in stomach cancer. Stored potatoes are similarly risky. To take just one example, in pregnant women who consume large amounts of potatoes, two mycotoxins produced by fungi commonly found in potatoes have been incriminated as a cause of spinal bifida in their offspring.

YEAST

You must eliminate all yeast products. We'll go over yeast in more detail in a later chapter. Here we're going to talk about eliminating brewer's yeast, baker's yeast and foods containing yeast in your diet.

You want to avoid taking in pure microforms. The most common ways to get yeast are bad for you for other reasons too. Beer and wine are double whammies as alcohol is harmful to your body in many ways. Breads and baked goods are a triple whammy because of the stored grains the flour is made from and the sugars and the other simple carbohydrates they contain. Eating yeast and anything made with yeast can spur microform overgrowth and increase mycotoxins, which increases the amount created in your own body in addition to whatever is in the product itself.

If you need anything else to discourage the use of products containing yeast, you should know that yeast food products could cause kidney stones and stones in the liver, gall bladder and even the brain; bone deposits, osteoarthritis, rheumatoid arthritis, kidney disease, heart disease, diabetes. In a 1990 study all mice fed a diet containing 10% brewer's yeast developed diabetes. It has also been linked to Sarcoidosis and auto immune diseases affecting the lungs, eyes and skin, Cirrhosis , and many cancers (particularly breast, prostate and liver cancer). Other resulting symptoms include Crone's disease and colitis.

Read labels carefully to make sure all foods, condiments and seasonings are yeast free.

EDIBLE FUNGUS

Mushrooms of all kinds and in all forms are all themselves the fruiting bodies of yeast or fungus, and form acids as they are digested. They also contain mycotoxins that poison human cells and lead to degenerative disease. Relatively speaking, there is no such thing as a good mushroom. The edible ones are just less poisonous than the ones that kill you immediately. Don't eat them. Don't drink them. Don't sniff them. Mushrooms all contain various amounts of mycotoxins and amanitin , which in large amounts will kill you almost instantly. With smaller amounts the result is the same, it just takes a little longer.

In a 1979 study, a leading cancer researcher administered mushroom mycotoxins to mice in their drinking water. She noted 21 different types of cancer as a result. We all know all mushrooms contain at least five active ingredients that exhibit carcinogenic properties in animals. Many impressive health claims have been made for some mushrooms but they do have occasional toxic side effects and all the same problems as any other mushroom.

FERMENTED AND MALTED PRODCUTS

This group includes condiments such as vinegar, mustard, ketchup, steak sauce, soy sauce, tamari, mayonnaise, salad dressing, chili sauce, horseradish, miso, monosodium glutamate (MSG) and any kind of alcohol, as well as pickled vegetables such as relish, green olives, sauerkraut and of course pickles and tempeh. All these are acid forming foods and create sticky mucus and with the exception of MSG are fermented by fungus.

Malt products such as malted milk and certain cereals or candies are also fermented by fungus. Besides containing high levels of sugar, malt products are acid forming and create sticky mucus.

ALCOHOL

It may help to think of alcohol as the mycotoxin made by the yeast that it is. That includes wine, beer, whiskey, brandy, gin, rum, and vodka; just to name the most popular. You already know alcohol abuse causes disease including cirrhosis of the liver, brain damage, cancer, fetal injury and death. That's before you factor in the damage any mycotoxin can do.

It doesn't take what mainstream medicine considers abusive quantities of alcohol for serious harm to be done. On top of that, the liver can convert alcohol into yet another mycotoxin, acetylaldehyde , with its own harmful ways.

CORN, CORN PRODUCTS, PEANUTS
and PEANUT PRODUCTS

Corn contains 25% micro toxin producing fungi, including recognized carcinogens. Peanuts contain 26%. On top of that, broken and ground nuts of any kind are really targets for airborne mold spores and quickly become rancid. You can see it on the nuts as dark or black discoloring. Contamination occurs during the growing process because the plants themselves are not resistant. Humans who eventually ingest them are also eating the fungi and their toxic waste, inoculating their digestive track with negative microforms.

Research has linked corn consumption with cancers of the esophagus and the stomach and peanuts with pancreatic and liver cancer. Cashew nuts and dried coconut are easily contaminated and should also be avoided. This is why raw nuts and seeds are preferred.

HEATED OILS

Any oils that have been cooked or heated in processing have

been nutritionally destroyed including the biggest brands of corn, canola and other vegetable oils. Look for cold pressed virgin oils instead, such as many olive oils. Choose from the healthy varieties, of course. Try to get first pressed, cold pressed olive oil.

MICROWAVED FOODS

First of all, microwaving your food destroys enzymes, depleting the life energy as foods are cooked, but it gets much worse. The Russians, who have done the most diligent research on microwave ovens and the biological effects on food and humans outlawed their use. In their research, foods that were exposed to microwave energy increased cancer causing effects and decreased nutritional value; vitamins and minerals were made useless in every food tested and their bio-availability of nutrients, including the B-Vitamins, Vitamin C and E, and essential minerals decreased; and meat proteins were rendered worthless.

Microwaving also interfered with the digestibility of fruits and vegetables. To top it all off, microwaving makes all foods acid forming. A higher than normal percentage of abnormal blood cells in the blood of people who ate microwave foods was also observed.

THE DIGESTIVE SYSTEM

Now that we have covered harmful toxins that are contained in most American diets, let's take a look at our digestive systems and how the foods we eat play a role in our overall health.

Degeneration is the gradual deterioration of specific tissues, cells or organs with corresponding impairment or loss of function caused by injury, disease or aging. Most professionals agree that degenerative diseases are preventable. Many believe that some of the degenerative conditions are reversible if severe damage has not been done.

There are many factors that contribute to degeneration, such as improper diet and nutrition, inadequate exercise, rest and water amounts and excessive toxins. The automobile is the perfect example to illustrate what happens when the wrong ingredients are added to a working machine. If one were to put sand in the gas tank and sugar in the engine, the automobile would be ruined in a very short time.

Our bodies work in the same manner. Fortunately our bodies are a little more forgiving; however, many people abuse the fact that our bodies are so forgiving by not taking care of their health. Degenerative diseases are earned from a lifetime of abuse.

Digestion disengages vitamins, minerals and other nutrients within food while breaking down carbohydrates, fats and proteins to smaller usable molecules. Carbohydrates and fats are fuel sources. Proteins can be used for fuel but are usually used for reconstruction within the body. Enzymes are responsible for breaking down food. If food is not in its most basic form (amino acids, monosaccharides , small polysaccharides , and fatty acids) when it enters the blood stream, the body will identify these large molecules as foreign bodies; thus causing an immune response. Incomplete digestion also prevents vitamins, minerals and other nutrients from being separated from the food, therefore rendering them useless.

Ironically enough, enzymes require vitamins, minerals and nutrients in order to function. Gas, bloating, indigestion, heartburn and other digestion discomforts can be due to improper break down of food. Enzymes are easily destroyed. Heat, storage, pesticides, chemicals and genetic engineering all leave enzymes worthless, forcing your body to produce enzymes when your food is devoid of them.

DIGESTIVE ENZYMES

If the food one eats does not contain digestive enzymes, the body is called upon to provide the digestive enzymes organically. In this instance, it is possible to overwork the digestive system. When this occurs, there are dire consequences. The consequences of an overworked digestive system include impaired liver and pancreas; digestive disorders including heartburn, indigestion, gas, bloating, constipation, diarrhea, and insomnia; improper food digestion; inadequate absorption of vitamins, minerals and other nutrients; immune response. It affects having symptoms such as allergies, arthritis, improper elimination of food, colon cancer.

What are enzymes? Enzymes are specialized proteins that catalyze every reaction in the body. Without enzymes, none of the body's systems would operate, including metabolism, elimination, digestion, reproduction, and gas exchange. There are many types of enzymes that are specific in their function. Enzymes required for the digestion of foods are called digestive enzymes. Solutions4 makes an amazing digestive enzyme and that will be covered further in Chapter Ten entitled "Supplements".

The food we eat is composed of three metabolites; carbohydrates, fats and proteins. In order for the body to utilize these metabolites, they must be digested to their most basic form. For example, proteins need to be broken down into polypeptides and amino acids.

There are four main types of digestive enzymes--amylase, protease, lipase and cellulase. Amylase breaks down carbohydrates. Protease breaks down proteins. Lipase breaks down fats. Cellulase breaks down cellulose. Humans do not produce this digestive enzyme. There are three sources for digestive enzymes: Fresh unaltered foods, our digestive system and the Solutions4 digestive enzyme supplement.

There are digestive enzymes found naturally in foods. However, these enzymes are very sensitive and easily destroyed. Food that is altered in any way is devoid of digestive enzymes and is considered dead. Heating foods to or above 118 degrees Fahrenheit, storage, pesticides, chemicals, hybridization, genetic engineering and pasteurization are some ways that enzymes are destroyed. You can either eat dead food or live food.

LIVER AND PANCREAS

The main digestive organs, the liver and pancreas, have functions other than digestion which make them very important organs. Over-taxation of the digestive system as a whole can lead to many degenerative diseases and obesity. The average American diet today is extremely demanding of the digestive system. This is due to most of our foods being cooked, processed, and consisting of material that is difficult for the body to digest, like grains, saturated or hydrogenated fats, large sugar molecules and dairy.

The liver and pancreas are two digestive organs that have other functions as well. The liver detoxifies the blood and helps regulate the metabolism. The pancreas helps regulate the metabolism and plays a vital role in the delicate endocrine system, which is the hormone system.

The consequences of a compromised liver are impaired blood purification, which causes oxidation reaction, free radicals, autoimmune disease, chronic fatigue syndrome, premenstrual syndrome, irritable bowel syndrome, inhibits the gall bladder, impairs bile secretion, improper fat digestion (which just ends up on the body), impairs metabolism regulation, enlarges the liver, reduces blood flow to pelvic and abdominal regions, causes hemorrhoids, bowel irritation, uterine, ovarian and prostate irritation, neck pain and stiffness; and in severe cases heart palpitations.

WHAT SHOULD WE EAT?
FACTS ABOUT PROTEIN

Studies show that protein from non meat sources such as almonds, sesame seeds, soy beans, buckwheat, peanuts, sunflower seeds, pumpkin seeds, potatoes and all leafy green vegetables are incomplete proteins, yet when consumed in a variety, can give the body the building blocks of amino acids for function and repair. In addition, these alternative sources of protein only require half as much protein to meet the body's needs when compared to animal sources. We need 30 to 60 grams of protein daily depending on the demand we put our physical body through like exercise. Pregnant or lactating women require about double this amount. Raw protein is utilized by the body twice as well as cooked protein, making these natural alternative sources of protein one of the healthiest choices you can make.

There are many dangers in over consuming protein. Research at the US Army Medical Research Lab in Denver, Colorado showed that the more meat one consumes, the more deficient they are in vitamin B-6, B-3, Magnesium, and calcium.

Extensive studies in England showed a clear connection between high protein diet and osteoporosis. Studies at the Vascular Research Laboratory in Brooklyn, New York concluded that excessive meat consumption causes atherosclerosis and heart disease. Studies at Cornell University linked a high protein diet to the development of cancer.

Ammonia is produced in great amounts as a by-product of meat metabolism. Ammonia is carcinogenic and can trigger cancer development. A high protein diet has been found to break down the pancreas and contribute to diabetes and hypoglycemia. The Max Plank Institute for Nutritional Research in Germany found that meat proteins leave toxic residues of metabolic waste in the tissues, causing auto toxemia, over acidity, nutritional deficiencies, accumulation of uric acid, intestinal putrefaction and leads to many diseases. Some of these would include arthritis, kidney damage, schizophrenia, osteoporosis, arterial sclerosis, heart disease and cancer. It is also noted that an over acidic body, due to too much protein, can cause obesity. They also found that a high protein diet causes premature aging and lowers life expectancy.

Where do you get your protein? For many people, the protein in their diet comes primarily only from meat, dairy and eggs. The truth is there is plenty of protein in plants and other sources. If you're getting enough calories to be healthy and you are eating a reasonable variety of foods, you're getting enough protein. A clinical study published in the Journal of American Dietetic Association analyzed the diets of all meat eaters; vegetarians who eat dairy and eggs and pure vegan vegetarians using strict requirements about how much protein would easily cover the requirements of growing children and pregnant women.

Not only did all three diets provide enough protein, but they actually doubled the daily protein requirements. The take-home message is no one has to worry about getting enough protein. If you eat a normal amount of reasonable food you will easily meet the daily requirements. Most people seem to think protein needs to come from meat and dairy products. Even those more in the know about alternative health subscribed for a long time to the theory that vegetable proteins are somehow second class and require proper combining to be complete. However, vegetables carry all the amino acids, the building blocks of protein, the body needs.

If you eat a wide variety of vegetables, especially dark green and dark green leafy vegetables, and supplement with grasses, you are getting plenty of all the essential amino acids. The body has a free amino acid pool which contributes about 70 grams of protein daily. We all have these protein reserves. So unless you have specific symptoms of protein deficiency (muscle tissue loss, hair falling out, brittle nails) you can be sure you're getting enough protein. The key to providing your body with protein is quality, not quantity.

JUICING

Juicing is the perfect tool to restore health and prevent disease. During the time of restoring health and for preventative measures, it makes sense to allow the digestive system to rest. When juicing fruits or vegetables, the fiber is separated from the nutrients and water allowing the body to receive the healing properties of food in a short amount of time because it can enter the blood stream directly while resting the digestive system.

Resting the digestive system gives the body an opportunity to focus its energy toward healing the body. The nutrition juice provides the body is invaluable. Enzymes are in a fresh, raw fruit and vegetable juice--as well as vitamins, minerals and other nutrients. Other properties and nutrients of juice are being continually found. It is suspected that researchers will continue to find attributes concerning whole foods and probably never find others because nutrients are added to multivitamins and multiminerals only after they are discovered, studied and deemed useful; and it is quite possible that there are nutrients unique to untreated wholesome vegetables and fruit juices.

Another redeeming quality of fresh juice is the composition and arrangement of nutrients that allow the body to maximize absorption and utilization of them. Canned, bottled and frozen juices do not have the nutrient and therapeutic value that fresh juices have. Not only do most of them contain too much sugar, but the process they have gone through to become bottled, canned or frozen has stripped them of their natural vitamins, minerals, enzymes and other nutrients by way of heating, storage and being treated with chemicals.

Organic, unwaxed, fresh raw fruits and vegetables are the most ideal to use for juicing. If these are not available, you must thoroughly wash the produce. The simplest method we've found for this is to simply fill your sink with cold water; add a few tablespoons of salt and the juice of half a lemon. Soak the produce for approximately ten minutes, then rinse. There is also the possibility of buying a natural commercial produce cleanser. For fruits that are commonly waxed, such as apples, it is recommended that you dip the fruit into boiling water for five seconds and lift it out of the water with tongs.

Different juices yield different results. The basic varieties are as follows.

FRUIT - Fruit juices are generally thought of as cleansing, refreshing and they offer a quick burst of energy. The high water content flushes the digestive track and kidneys as well as purifies the blood stream. Grapes, apples and lemons are all strong purifiers. Fruit juices are high in sugars. Although these sugars are natural, the amount you drink should be modified, especially those who have been advised to limit sugar consumption.

CARROT and CARROT COMBINATIONS - Carrot juice is generally thought of as being an energy drink. Carrot juice is sweet so it's often recommended to mix carrots with other vegetables to cut back on sweets. When you're making carrot combination juices, the carrot proportion should always dominate. Unless they're organic carrots, they should be trimmed about one half inch from the green because that's where pesticides are concentrated. Organic carrots do not need to be trimmed, just washed.

GREEN JUICES - This is what is thought of as "serious" juice. Green juices are healing, stabilizing and calming. The energy they offer is centering. They are best enjoyed in the evening. Green juices are a potent cocktail of nutrition. Because green juices are so powerful unless they are diluted with carrot or apple juice, they can cause lightheadedness and gastric distress . Only about a quarter of your glass should be green juice, with the rest being carrot, apple or a combination of the two. Vegetables that can be used for green juices are alfalfa sprouts, barley greens, cabbage, kale, dandelion greens, green chard, lettuce varieties, parsley, spinach and wheat grass.

THE "UNJUICEABLES" - These fruits and vegetables yield so little water that at best they can leave you with very little to drink and at worst they can damage your juicer. Avoid juicing apricots, avocado, bananas, blueberries, cantaloupe, coconut, honeydew melon, papaya, peaches, plums, prunes, or strawberries. When you see commercial juices with any of the above ingredients, it is usually the pulp of the fruit mixed with a lot of apple or grape juice.

It is best to wash and chop your produce right before juicing and to drink it right after juicing. Otherwise your juice rapidly loses nutritional potency. While it is best to drink juices right after they're made, they should be slowly sipped rather than gulped. Oranges, tangerines and grapefruits should be peeled before juicing, but use a vegetable peeler so as to just remove the rind, not the nutrient-rich white covering the food known as pith. These particular fruits should be peeled because their skins contain toxic substances and are also bitter. Apple seeds contain some cyanide, so it is recommended that they are removed.

When you're making vegetable juice that contains produce with a strong odor like garlic and ginger, the stronger smelling items should be among the first to be juiced. This ensures that the ones that follow can push the last remains through. Because of digestion considerations, fruits and vegetables generally do not mix together with the exception of apples and carrots.

Like herbs, juices are specific to the organs they strengthen and conditions they are used for. The following is a list of these.

Lemons: liver, gall bladder, allergies, asthma, cardiovascular disease and colds.

Citrus: Obesity, hemorrhoids, and varicose veins.

Apples: liver and intestines.

Pears: gall bladder.

Grapes: colon and anemia.

Papaya: stomach health, indigestion, hemorrhoids, and

colitis.

Pineapple: allergies, arthritis, inflammation, edema, hemorrhoids.

 Watermelon: Kidneys, edema.

Black Cherry: Colon, menstrual problems, gout.

Greens: Skin, eczema, digestive problems, obesity, breath.

Spinach: Anemia, eczema.

Parsley: Kidney, edema, arthritis.

Beet greens: Gall bladder, liver, osteoporosis.

Water Cress: Anemia, colds.

Wheat Grass: Anemia, liver, intestines, breath.

Cabbage: Colitis, ulcer.

Comfrey: Intestines, hypertension, osteoporosis.

Carrots: Eyes, arthritis, osteoporosis.

Beets: Blood, liver, menstrual problems, Arthritis.

Celery: Kidneys, diabetes, osteoporosis.

Cucumber: Edema, diabetes.

Jerusalem Artichokes: Diabetes.

Garlic: Allergies, colds, hypertension, high fats, diabetes.

Radish: Liver, high fats, obesity.

Potatoes: Intestines, ulcer.

While these examples are helpful in some of these conditions, they are not meant to cure disease. These are given for preventive measures only.

A final word about juicing for improved health. Raw, fresh juices are rich in vitamins, minerals and enzymes. Almost 100% of the vital nutrients go directly into the blood stream. Thus, the blood carries it to the muscles and tissues and heals the body. The best juices for therapeutic purposes are fresh, raw, natural juices prepared in your own juicer immediately before drinking.

In the form of juice, a greater amount of vegetables can be taken into the system than could possibly be eaten. These juices build strong and healthy cells. Thus, the body can be revitalized in an amazingly short time. If your juice is very sweet, dilute it 50/50 with pure water. This is very important for Fibroidmyalgia, arthritis, diabetes, hypoglycemia, and high blood pressure. Remember, the fresher the juice the greater the nutrition.

JUICING RECIPES FOR WEIGHT LOSS

Energy Shake
Handful Parsley
4-6 Carrots, greens removed
Parsley sprig for garnish

Bunch up parsley and push through hopper with carrots. Garnish with sprig of parsley.

Ginger Hopper
¼ in. slice ginger root
4-5 carrots, greens removed
½ apple, seeded

Push ginger through hopper with carrots and apple.
Pink Morning Tonic

1 pink grapefruit peeled, leaving white pithy part
1 red delicious apple, seeded
Push grapefruit through hopper with apple.
Zippy Spring Tonic
Handful dandelion greens, unsprayed
3 pineapple rings with skin
3 radishes

Bunch up dandelion greens and push through hopper with pineapple and radishes.

Potassium Broth
Handful parsley
Handful spinach
4-5 carrots, greens removed
2 stalks celery

Bunch up parsley and spinach leaves and push through hopper with carrots and celery.

Berry Cantaloupe shake
Half cantaloupe with skin
5-6 strawberries

Push cantaloupe and strawberries through hopper.
Garden Salad Special

> 3 broccoli florets
> 1 garlic clove
> 4-5 carrots or 2 tomatoes
> 2 stalks celery
> ½ green pepper

Push broccoli and garlic through the hoppers and carrots or tomatoes. Follow with celery and green pepper.

> Spring Tonic
> Handful parsley
> 4 carrots, greens removed
> 1 garlic clove

Bunch up parsley and push through hopper with carrots, garlic and celery.

ACID VERSUS ALKALINE FOODS

When foods are metabolized in the body they become either alkaline or acidic. Some foods that taste acidic break down in the digestive system to become alkaline for the body. For example, citrus fruits are alkaline once they are metabolized.

Our bodies are slightly alkaline and the majority of our diets should consist of alkaline or balanced foods. Acidic foods are also called mucus forming because when they are metabolized they form mucus within the body. When one's diet is mainly acidic or one's body does not tolerate acidic foods, mucus is secreted out of the body. This function helps the body to regain an alkaline environment. An alkaline environment will reinforce the detoxification process.

Lemon is used to detoxify the body because of many properties it has. Lemon contains digestive enzymes and is considered a predigested food, which rests the digestive system. It contains vitamins and minerals which help to provide the body with complete nutrition, leaves alkaline residues in the body when metabolized, which supports the detoxification process and helps maintain the body's slightly alkaline environment. Lemon juice is an excellent cleansing agent.

Some examples of alkaline foods include avocado, corn, dates, fresh coconut, fresh fruits, fresh vegetables, honey, horseradish, maple syrup, molasses, mushrooms, onions, raisins, soy products, sprouts, plums*, watercress.

Low level alkaline foods include almonds, blackstrap molasses, Brazil nuts, chestnuts, lima beans, millet.

Acid foods include alcohol, asparagus, beans, Brussels sprouts, buckwheat, catnip, ketchup, chick peas, cocoa, coffee, cornstarch, cranberries, most drugs, eggs, fish, flour, legumes, lentils, meat, milk, mustard, noodles, oatmeal, olives, organ meats, pasta, pepper, plums*, poultry, prunes, sauerkraut, shellfish, soft drinks, sugar, tea, vinegar.

*This food leaves an alkaline ash but has an acidifying effect on the body.

Although it might seem that citrus fruits would have an acidifying effect on the body, the citric acid they contain actually has an alkalinizing effect in the system. Foods acid or alkaline forming tendency in the body has nothing to do with the actual acidic level (ph) of the food itself. Lemons are very acidic; however the end products they produce after digestion and assimilation are very alkaline, so lemons are alkaline forming in the body. Likewise meat will test alkaline before digestion, but it leaves acidic residue in the body like nearly all animal products. Meat is very acid forming causing more harm to the body if consumed in over abundance.

MORE ON WATER

Are you thirsty? Everything we do on a consistent basis sends a signal to our bodies, and the body in turn reacts to that signal. The result may be a healthy reaction or an unhealthy reaction. The inner communication with our bodies is a two way system. By this we send signals to the body and the body also sends signals to us. The body tells us when it is tired and hopefully we sleep. The body tells us when we have had an injury through the sensation of pain and hopefully we listen to the signal and address the problem. However, there is one need we consistently overlook or misinterpret the signals for. That need is water.

What is water? We are all aware of water in the most basic sense. As defined by Webster's Dictionary water is the colorless transparent liquid occurring on earth as rivers, lakes, oceans, and falling from the clouds as rain. It is chemically a compound of oxygen and hydrogen, H2O, and under laboratory conditions it freezes hard, forming ice at 32 degrees Fahrenheit and boils, forming steam, at 212 degrees Fahrenheit.

Based on this definition, water sounds as if it is a fairly uncomplicated, if not somewhat boring aspect of nature. However, water is truly a miracle substance. Water accounts for nearly 70% of our world, 70-75% of our bodies. Obviously water plays a large part of our survival and is one of the greatest necessities to the continuation of life.

How important is Water? It is one of the four main items necessary for human survival. Those necessities are air, water, sleep and food (in order of importance). When deprived of air, the human life span can be measured in a matter of minutes. As you can see from the above list, water came second only to air as a basic human need. Without water in some form humans cannot survive much longer than one week. This time frame can vary depending on a person's location. If you're in a drier or warmer climate such as desert, the dehydration will occur much sooner and the risk of fatality will increase significantly as opposed to a more humid climate.

How does this affect us? Most of us are aware of the dangers of being stranded in a desert with no fresh water. In reality, the chances of this happening are very slim. Only 1 to 2% of the population will ever find themselves in such a predicament. It is much easier to become dehydrated than most people realize. The truth is that if you're thirsty right now then you are already dehydrated. Every part of the body depends on water to function properly. With everything we do we are depleting our resources. As our water reserves are used, the body sends signals telling us what it needs. Thirst is one of the last and most obvious signals from the body. There are many other signals that we ignore or do not understand.

Am I thirsty? One of the most common ways in which we misinterpret our need for water is mistaking it for hunger. Before eating, drink an eight ounce glass of water and wait five minutes. Chances are you were only thirsty. This common mistake is one of the greatest contributing factors to overeating and weight problems.

Have a headache? Next time you feel a headache coming on, don't necessarily run for the bottle of Tylenol or ibuprofen. Those drugs do not cure the headache. They only treat the symptom temporarily. Rather than using a quick fix, look to the root of the problem. You're probably dehydrated. The brain's tissue consists of 85% water. With such a high dependency on water, it is very easy for the brain to become dehydrated. This heat stress can be brought about in several different ways. Excessive bed covers will limit your body's ability to breathe and regulate its temperature, contributing to dehydration. A more obvious cause is exercise, especially in extreme heat. This dehydration triggers headaches and is also the number one cause of memory loss.

Is all water created equal? The simple answer to this is no.

There are nine different types of water. Some can cause hardening of the arteries, gall stones, kidney stones, and the onset of early senility.

One type of water is hard water. This water is dangerous to our health. Hard water contains all the vital minerals but also contains other substances such as viruses, chemicals and other inorganic substances. Raw water is water that has not been treated in any way. Every type of this type of water is densely inhabited by millions of viruses and bacteria. Boiled water is not the answer. You may be able to kill the millions of microorganisms, germs and bacteria, but now you're left with a full glass of dead organisms. You can say you're drinking a graveyard of microorganisms. Rain water is actually distilled water that passes through the atmosphere of the earth. Due to the filth and pollutants in the air, this water becomes polluted and needless to say this is not good for our bodies and can cause cancer and other serious side effects. Snow water is rain water that has frozen. The cold doesn't kill the germs, so you basically have the same effect as the rain water.

Filtered water is water that has passed through a filter or a very fine strainer. Many chemicals are removed but there is no filtering system that can assure that all the bacteria are removed unless the water is completely stripped. Some filtration systems actually cause bacteria to form. Without chlorine, this water can become a breeding ground. Deionized water is water comparable to distilled water, except it does not remove chemicals such as herbicides, pesticides, insecticides or industrial solvents. The stipulation for bottled water is that it must be as good as city water or tap water. The one difference is that the chlorine is removed. However, once the chlorine is removed, now there is nothing left to battle the germs and bacteria. If you currently drink bottled water you have taken the first step in realizing that common drinking water is not the answer.

Distilled water is how nature intended water to be. Natured designed the perfect distillation unit. When water is heated it becomes a gas. It is completely stripped of harmful germs and bacteria. When this gas is trapped the liquid that is produced is pure H2O. Adding minerals back into this water is the final step. Water is the ultimate replenishment for mind, body and spirit. Pure water is essential for survival and by drinking at least half one's body weight in ounces per day we may be able to prevent the need for our bodies to send any uncomfortable reminders.

VEGETABLES

Vegetables should be the focus of your diet; the majority of any meal you sit down to; the substance covering most of your plate. You want to look at vegetables as your new best friends. They are the lowest calorie, lowest sugar, most nutrient-rich foods on the planet. Beyond that, they provide vitamins, minerals, fiber, chlorophyll, enzymes, phytonutrients and alkaline salts that control microforms and their micro toxins.

Choose from a variety of vegetables, making the majority of them green. Vegetables are an excellent source of the alkaline salts that protect against microform overgrowth as well as help to neutralize acids in the blood and tissue. Fresh is essential. Organically grown is preferable.

A vegetable's green color is produced by chlorophyll, sometimes referred to as the blood of plants, because the molecular structure and chemical components are similar to that of human blood. Chlorophyll helps the blood cells deliver oxygen throughout the body. It also reduces the binding of carcinogens to DNA in the liver and other organs. If that is not enough of a benefit for you, keep in mind that it also breaks down calcium stones; stones that the body creates to neutralize and dispose of excess acid for elimination. Green vegetables, particularly leafy greens, have the highest amounts of chlorophyll.

Vegetables and particularly green vegetables are incredibly nutrient dense and provide just about all the vitamins and minerals and micronutrients you could ever need. Vegetables are loaded with the fiber that is crucial to your diet. Besides the accepted benefits of fiber in reducing cancer and other serious health concerns, studies have shown that fiber markedly decreases micro-toxicity. Fiber acts like a sponge soaking up acids from the body. It also works like a broom cleaning out the intestines. Vegetables are plentiful sources of the enzymes that are needed for just about every chemical activity in the human body.

Among other things, the enzymes in vegetables aid in proper digestion. Different enzymes are called upon according to the foods eaten and how it was processed. Whatever the enzymes within the food can accomplish in the way of digestion makes less work for the digestive enzymes of the body. Again, heat over 118 degrees destroys enzymes, which is why you want to get a lot of your food uncooked or at least cooked as little time as possible. Cooked food requires the body to produce all the necessary enzymes, creating unnecessary stress and diverting resources from other jobs.

GRASSES

Grasses are incredibly nutrient dense, even more so than vegetables. It is a good idea to look for a wide variety of grasses such as wheat grass, barley grass, oat grass, dog grass, camut grass, lemongrass and shave grass. It's best to avoid all algae and mushrooms.

Wheat grass and barley grass are particularly good sources of chlorophyll and it is the chlorophyll that gives grasses the power to regenerate our bodies at the molecular and cellular level. To give you just two examples, wheat grass contains more than 100 food elements, including every identified mineral and trace mineral and every vitamin in the B complex family. It has one of the highest pro vitamin A contents of any food. It is rich in vitamins C, E, and K.

Wheat grass juice is 25% protein, a higher percentage than in meat, fish, eggs, dairy products and beans. In addition, it has high amounts of an antifungal, antimycotoxic substance called laetrile. Barley grass boasts four times as much thiamine, B1, as whole flour and thirty times as much as milk. It has seven times more vitamin C than an orange.

RAW FOODS

Since cooking destroys those all important enzymes, the more of your vegetables you eat raw, the better. Aim to have at least 40%, visually, of your food uncooked, working up to 75-80%. Think salads, great big salads, in infinite variety. Raw foods also contain energy or life force, which they transfer to you, while cooked foods are dead.

WHERE DO WE GO FROM HERE?

As you can see from this chapter, an acidic diet rich in caffeine, sugar, hydrogenated fats and other chemicals is disease forming. An alkaline diet containing fresh fruits, vegetables and healthy proteins is health producing. To find out more, we have various programs available to you to give you instructions on foods, menu plans, recipes, what to put together to feed you and your family that will give you health, energy, the sleep; and yes, the weight loss that you desire.

Cancer cells feed on sugar and any artificial sweeteners as well, like milk, causing the body to produce mucus, especially in the gastrointestinal tract. Cancer feeds on mucus. Cells thrive in an acidic environment. A meat based diet is acidic. It is better to eat fish and a little chicken rather than beef or pork, not to mention the livestock and animals contain antibiotics, growth hormone and parasites all of which are harmful. A diet of 80% fresh vegetables and juices along with raw nuts and seeds can put your body into an alkaline environment. 10-20% can be fruits; seasonal fruits. There is a specific nutritional program we, at Club Reduce®, can put you on according to your results and needs determined in the Symptom Survey.

CHAPTER

THREE

Detoxification

DETOXIFICATION

We learned in the previous chapter that the foods we eat are inundating our bodies with toxic chemicals and harmful substances that can cause chronic health problems and disease. To rid our bodies of these harmful substances cleansing internally is extremely important. Detoxification is the metabolic process by which the toxic qualities of a poison or toxin are reduced by the body. Detoxification is the foundation of all of our programs at Club Reduce. Almost every chronic disease is due to the influence of bacterial poisons diffusing into the body systems from the intestine. 95% of all degenerative disease begins in the colon. Detoxification is the process of total body cleansing. It cleanses the liver, bowels, kidneys, blood supply and tissues, helps to restore the peristaltic action to the colon. It cleanses mucus, toxins, waste material from our bodies.

Some of the symptoms which signal the need to detoxify are things like lack of energy; overweight; mental confusion; allergies; eliminating less than twice daily; dependency on sugar, caffeine, alcohol, drugs; bad skin; body odor; excessive perspiration; headaches; and digestive irregularity.

SIGNS OF A TOXIC BODY

Is your body toxic? How would you know? Some signs of a toxic body include mental confusion, mood swings, anxiety, depression, irritability, overweight, fatigue, lack of energy, insomnia, stress, headaches, cravings or addictions, digestive problems, allergies, hay fever, asthma, male or female problems, PMS, prostate issues, hot flashes, impotence, infertility, low libido, eating disorders--anorexia, bulimia, excessive appetite; low resistance to illness and infection, life threatening and degenerative illness, bowel irregularity, painful inflammation, yeast infections, strong desires for sugar, beer, bread, high risk of coronary artery disease, diabetes or hypoglycemia, high blood pressure, skin disorders, acne, eczema, psoriasis, weakness, shakiness, poor muscle tone, muscle soreness or spasm, high alcohol consumption, high caffeine consumption and smoking. Many of these symptoms and signs of a toxic body are also signs and symptoms of Candida, which we'll cover in another chapter.

Our bodies retain fat because fat cells envelop toxins. The more toxins in a fat cell, the larger the fat cell will grow. We create a finite number of fat cells up until puberty. After puberty we don't grow new fat cells. The fat cells we have just get larger.

THE ELIMINATING AND CLEANSING ORGANS

The colon is the large intestine that acts as the disposal for human body waste. Most of what we eat, breathe, drink and anything our body is trying to slough off such as atrophied tissue, dead cell growth, is eliminated through the colon. This organ performs the peristaltic action to move the waste along for elimination. The entire process of elimination should take twenty four to thirty six hours; however, because of poor lifestyle an individual's track time may be six to thirty days, which leads to the colon becoming clogged with waste. This forms layers of encrustation on its walls. The encrusted waste material begins decomposing and causes fermentation and putrefaction leading to disease. The eliminative organ, also known as the intestines, is the final step in digesting the foods that we eat. This process starts in your mouth and the stomach and ends up when you go to the bathroom. Toxic waste is eliminated by diarrhea, dark heavy stools, parasites, worms, old fecal material.

The skin is the largest organ of the body. Its functions are protection and body temperature regulation. It iis the largest organ that excretes waste from the body. Elimination of waste materials is by perspiration.

The lungs are a pair of sponge-like organs in the chest which are primarily responsible for the exchange of oxygen and carbon dioxide between the air we breathe and the blood. The lungs also eliminate mucus through coughing and a runny nose.

The kidneys regulate the body's fluid volume, mineral composition and acidity. Toxins are eliminated through urine. The liver may be the most important organ of the body for supporting overall physical health. It is best known for its role in detoxification, transforming harmful substances like ammonia, metabolic waste, drugs and chemicals so that they may be excreted. It is also the source of bile which breaks down fat.

During a detoxification cleansing program, the lymphatic system is also cleansed. The immune system's own circulatory system, it permeates every organ of the body except the brain. It is called the river of life; has more mileage than the circulatory system; sweeps toxins, bacteria, virus, germs, mutant cells and harmful substances away from the body; carries destructive substances away in the lymph through the thoracic valve of the heart, then reenters the blood stream to be purified by the liver and eliminated by the kidneys.

If lymphatic flow is weak the virus, toxins, bacteria, et cetera cannot be completely eliminated. The invader may reemerge and re-manifest itself, possibly as much as thirty to fifty years later. Water is very critical in this process.

Every organ of the body runs on water. You must continually cleanse your body with water to make every organ of the body responds and keeps well. As a reminder, you should drink at least one half your body weight in ounces of water each day.

CLEANSING 101

How do we rid our bodies of the toxins we ingest on a daily basis? Cleansing is the most effective way to detoxify the body naturally. In our office, any cleansing process begins with what we call a basic cleanse. The basic cleanse consists of a liquid diet comprised of a mixture of fresh lemon juice, distilled water and pure maple syrup.

We recommend that at least two quarts of lemon mixture are consumed each day. During the actual cleansing process no solid foods are allowed. The actual cleansing process ranges from three to ten days. Complete herbal formulas and a fiber supplement help to expedite cleansing.

Understand, a cleanse is not a three day fast. It merely substitutes a normal diet of food for one that will help cleanse the body. The body will get all the calories and nutrients it needs with the predigested lemon juice formula and the supplements we recommend, which we'll cover later on.

The first two days of the program are considered preparation days. During this time, you must eliminate meat, dairy, refined sugar and flour. Wean yourself off any abusive substances such as alcohol, tobacco and coffee; and again remember to drink at least half your body weight in ounces of distilled water daily.

After the two initial prep days, the cleanse moves on to days three, four and five; the three day detoxification process. These are the days you will revert to drinking your lemon juice concoction, while continuing to drink pure distilled water and take your supplements. Days six through twenty are considered the twenty day rejuvenation period in our office, where we build on the good work days one through six have accomplished.

WHAT'S IN A CLEANSE?

To prepare for the lemonade detox program, you will need twenty one fresh lemons, one pint of pure maple syrup and at least two gallons of distilled water. Combine one and a half cups fresh squeezed lemon juice, a third to a half cup of pure maple syrup grade A or B, and two quarts of distilled water to consume daily.

Lemon juice is rich in water soluble vitamins that the body cannot store. Pure maple syrup is a balanced form of natural sugar that won't cause an insulin response. Pure maple syrup is also rich in minerals that the body needs and also provides the calories needed for the body to function properly.

An individual can cleanse anywhere from three to ten days. You cannot detoxify if you are pregnant or nursing. If you are taking any prescription drugs you must continue to take these medications. Those under medical treatment should get approval from their doctor before beginning any program, specifically those suffering from cancer, epilepsy and heart conditions that require cumatin and related medications.

The benefits of doing this cleanse are numerous. It increases energy, rejuvenates the body, has anti aging benefits, helps clean out mucus, toxins and waste material, restores normal elimination, helps with liver, kidney and blood purification, achieves mental clarity, reduces dependency on drugs, helps restore the peristaltic action of the colon, and it's a very big step towards a healthier lifestyle. You can lose anywhere from three to eight pounds while breaking bad eating habits and starting to feel amazing.

THE HEALING CRISIS

During detoxification you may experience something called a healing crisis. This is a good thing. A healing crisis is when the body is eliminating toxins that have been stored for numerous years. There are a few symptoms that you may experience while you're cleansing. These include diarrhea, dark foul stools, dark urine, skin eruptions, coated tongue, foul breath, fatigue, irritability, anxiety, mucus discharge, coughing, poor concentration, confusion, headaches, joint or muscle pain, coughing, flu. You may feel that you're getting a fever. This is your body's way of natural cleansing.

Cleansing reactions can take up to a few hours to a few days. The healthier a person is the milder the healing crisis. The more the body has to clean up, the harder and longer and more difficult the healing crisis may be. Again, remember, the healing crisis is a positive event.

CELLULITE

What is cellulite? Cellulite is a toxic accumulation of fluid retention, poor circulation, poor lymphatic flow, lack of exercise, nutrient deficiency, and a toxic colon.

Cellulite is not actually fat. It's actually a toxic body condition combined with edema and lack of circulation. A person doesn't have to be overweight to have cellulite. Thin people are affected. Thin people can also have problems with toxins in the body which cause cellulite. Cellulite does not respond to normal exercise and weight loss programs, because it's not fat. Eight out of ten women have cellulite as well as many men.

Cellulite consists of uneven deposits of water and waste that have become trapped in the connective tissue just below the skin, in the subcutaneous fat. There is hard cellulite. This is where you can squeeze the skin and there is a ripple and it appears like an orange peel . Soft cellulite is more advanced. It shakes around a lot, slides easily over muscles, and ripple will be noticed without applying any pressure.

Certain foods contribute to cellulite including increased estrogen and hormonal activities, various drugs, excessive weight, crash dieting followed by weight gain, constipation, inadequate water intake, lack of exercise, cigarettes, excessive stress, genetic predisposition.

To help eliminate cellulite detoxification is very important. Lymphatic cleansing wraps that clean the internal waste system are also helpful. Both are addressed in our program. Detoxification is part of our cellulite program. It's going to cleanse the liquid waste systems of your body, cleanse the body's connective tissue to help eliminate waste materials, helps eliminate cellulite and helps to soften and break down toxins and waste products.

You can literally lose one half a dress size or pants size per treatment. Detoxification stimulates circulation to aid in healing areas of body due to poor circulation, such as the lower extremities for people who are diabetic and pre diabetic. It also reduces water retention and tightens and tones the skin. Detoxification is a critical part of any program, particularly in patients with Fibroidmyalgia, Candida, weight loss or any health issue that involves a depleted immune system.

BODY WRAPS

One of the things that we recommend for detoxification is a body wrap. These body wraps were developed by a biochemist from the UCLA Medical Center.

How does a body wrap work?

A body wrap works by ridding the body of toxins and dead skin cells. It also helps to unclog pores and treat body blemishes like acne. Most of the toxins and dead skin cells are removed during the exfoliation process as surface skin layers are sloughed off to remove healthier skin underneath. The application of the mask followed by the

45-minute wrap allow the body to fully absorb the nutrients such as vitamin E and antioxidants in the lotion. Some masks may also contain salicylic acid, particularly if the client suffers from acne. The client is left with glowing skin after the treatment.

Before each wrap you should always exfoliate the body and use a cream specifically for body wrapping. This cream will softens the waste, stimulate circulation and help to flush out waste through normal body function. Purification and elimination are the main goals for these wraps, not weight loss. These wraps are not a water loss wrap. The inches lost are permanent because of body cleansing. It is an internal cleansing process. The Niacin based cream that we recommend will promotes circulation. Niacin also is a nutrient that does not flush well from a toxic body. Niacin retention can cause a hive reaction, so we alternatively will use a sensitive skin cream to prevent any reaction. Such reactions are very rare.

DOS and DON'TS OF WRAPPING

DO Start taking the cellulite cleanse that we will review at the supplement chapter at least one week prior to starting the wrap series. DO drink a minimum of half your body weight in ounces of water at least each day, at least one week prior to receiving the first body wrap. Continue this habit forever.

DO ensure that you practice a healthy lifestyle, including your diet, to maintain the inches lost forever.

DO drink at least half your daily allotment of water before drinking anything else, but do not drink anything within an hour of receiving wrap so you do not need to go to the bathroom while wrapped. Do use the anti cellulite lotion each day after a bath or shower.

DO ensure that you perform some exfoliation at home with a scrub in the shower.

DO ensure that if you are sensitive to niacin that you are not using any tanning creams or vitamins that contain niacin two days prior to the wrap.

DO consider doing an internal detoxification program to

enhance cellulite and inch loss. That means to also do the cleansing detoxification three day or ten day lemonade purification program which will help with inch loss as well.

DO NOT allow yourself to be wrapped if you have a heart condition, conditions requiring cumata, epilepsy, have had cancer that is not in remission or are pregnant or nursing.

DO NOT use a lotion or cream the day of your wrap.

DO NOT shave the day of your wrap.

DO NOT consume carbonated drinks such as coffee, refined sugar drinks, white flour, red meat and do not shower within six to eight hours of receiving the wrap.

There are several types of competing wrap types including salt solutions, clay, seaweed, hot oil wraps. These types promote a poultice effect. Detoxifying and inch loss come from internally to externally through the pores as a hydration loss.

The body wraps that we perform at Club Reduce detoxify the skin, cleanses the lymphatic waste system, inch loss through tissue cleansing--four to fourteen inches per treatment--helps restore elasticity of the skin, feeds and nourishes the skin, increases circulation by dilating blood vessels, increases metabolic function with vitamin A.

While doing body wraps, we recommend a product called Cellulite Cleanse from Solutions4, as it helps to break down cellulite, eliminate waste materials, reduce water retention and increase circulation and it appeases the appetite naturally. Another product from Solutions4 that we recommend is exercise gel. This is a liquid that you rub on the body to keep muscles warm and mobile, increases circulation, expels toxic waste and fluids, helps produce inch loss in conjunction with exercise; and functions as an anti-cellulite lotion.

We feel these products are important to help maintain the concentration of active ingredients on the skin in order to continue cleansing and aid in cellulite removal, increase the circulation, soften and condition the skin, tighten and tone, enhance tanning in tanning beds, and leave the skin with a really great smelling cinnamon scent. Maintain anti cellulite lotion contains essential nutrients to help continue the contouring, toning and tightening process started by the body wraps from Solutions4. It is scientifically formulated to be used as a take-home follow-up lotion to a professional Solutions4 body contour wrap and for anybody involved in the Solutions4 inch loss program. Maintain anti cellulite lotion should be applied immediately after showering or bathing on the areas that you would like to have toned. On all days, in between body wraps, it may also be used as an everyday circulation lotion. Apply to dry skin in a circular motion treating the problem areas of the hips, buttocks, thighs, upper arms et cetera.

FREQUENTLY ASKED QUESTIONS ABOUT DETOXIFICATION

Q: *Is Detoxification safe?*
A: Absolutely. Body cleansing for health is a concept that has been used for thousands of years. This type of internal cleanse has been use safely for periods of up to two months over the last thirty years. Solutions4 recommends detoxification for three to ten days only, three to four times per year. See your health care practitioner for specific directions.

Q: *Can I detoxify if I have hypoglycemia?*
A: Detoxifying is especially beneficial to those with hypoglycemia. Just be sure to use only pure maple syrup in the lemon juice mixture. Honey or other sweeteners will trigger an unhealthy insulin response. Solutions4's appetite appeaser will also help to regulate blood sugar levels.

Q: *How does detoxification affect cellulite?*
A: Cellulite is waste material trapped in connective tissue and fat cells. It is very resistant to ordinary dieting and exercise. While detoxification will not remove cellulite, it does cleanse the intestinal track and the body's liquid waste system; thereby speeding up the elimination of toxins from the body, which aides in cellulite removal. Improved results can be achieved when done in conjunction with Solutions4 body contouring wraps.

Q: *Will I have energy during the cleanse?*
A: As toxins are expelled from the system, the energy levels rise. It may take a day or two for this effect to occur. If you are not as energetic as you feel you should be, add a little more maple syrup to the lemon juice mixture to raise and maintain your blood sugar levels. It is also helpful to make the mixture last throughout the day rather than drinking it all at once. Sip slowly. Hypoglycemics or diabetics especially should be drinking this liquid every ten minutes. Solutions4 recommends reducing physical activity on detoxification days.

Q: *Why is it important to use distilled water?*
A: Distilled water is pure, which means it has no chemicals or bacteria to interfere with the cleansing process. We recommend continuing to use distilled and/or pure spring water after your cleansing program. Do not use bottled mineral water since it may contain concentrations of heavy metals. Soft water is also poor choice because of its high sodium content.

Q: *Will I suffer hunger pains during detoxification?*
A: Yes, you might. If you do, simply drink the lemon juice mixture more often and make sure you're taking the Appetite Appeaser. Since this mixture is food already, in liquid form, it gets into the blood stream faster and always helps with your hunger. You might think you're hungry because you aren't chewing food, but the mixture you're getting has all the nutrients you need.

Q: *Why is it important to use pure maple syrup?*
A: Pure maple syrup contains many minerals and vitamins. For this reason it will provide the body with energy. Second, pure maple syrup is a balanced natural sweetener and can be used without causing an insulin response. Because of this, hypoglycemic can use the program without fear of lowering or raising blood sugar levels.

Q: *Won't the lemon juice mixture cause too much acid for my sensitive stomach?*

A: No. Even though lemon is an acid fruit, it turns alkaline as it is digested and aids in attaining a proper Ph balance. To further avoid extra acidity, alternate drinking water in the lemon detox mixture.

The foundation of all of our Solutions4 programs in the basic body cleanse includes a product, body purifier, intestinal cleanser and fiber blend. We'll go over these products in more depth in the supplement chapter; but to review what goes into the detoxification kit, first we'll cover the Body Purifier by Solutions4. Body Purifier helps the body remove congestion, mucus, chemicals, purifies the blood, cleanses the lymphatic system, fights bacteria, virus, yeast, mold and worms, restores energy, destroys parasites in the digestive system. The second product in the kit is the Intestinal Cleanser. This helps the body to increase circulation to the bowels, lubricate the intestinal track, relieve gas and pain, expel intestinal parasites, reduce inflammation and irritation in joints and intestinal track, and improves the function of the stomach and liver.

The third product is Fiber Blend. This overcomes constipation, cleanses the bowels, stimulates the natural actions of the intestine, protects from putrefaction or pathogenic bacteria, lowers cholesterol and triglyceride levels, aides diabetes, heart disease, gall bladder disorder, varicose veins, diverticulitis and appendicitis.

CHAPTER

FOUR

Symptoms – Candida

CHAPTER FOUR -
WHAT ARE YOUR SYMPTOMS TELLING YOU?
WEIGHT GAIN AND CANDIDA

If you were driving your car and the red engine light came on would you ignore it? No. If you were asleep at home and the fire alarm went off would you just, turn it off, and go back to sleep? No. But that's exactly what we do to our bodies. When we're tired, when we can't sleep, when we have low libido, when we have uncontrollable cravings, these are symptoms of a bigger problem, but we tend to ignore the symptoms and continue on with our lives as though nothing is wrong. These symptoms are trying to tell you something. Just like the fire alarm has a purpose, the symptoms you have are telling you something. Believe it or not, these symptoms can also be related to your stubborn weight gain. Your symptoms are trying to tell you something. They may be trying to tell you that you have Candida.

THE CLUB REDUCE SYMPTOM ASSESSMENT SCALE

How many of these symptoms do you have?
How are these symptoms disrupting your life and how severe?

At Club Reduce®, we have a questionnaire that we have patients fill out. There are symptom assessment questionnaires within every profession out there, but the questionnaire that we use in our office will help the doctors and other health practitioners to stop some early indicator warning signs and symptoms and start a patient on a good nutritional program that fits them. We're going to briefly review some of the questions in the symptom assessment over the next few pages. This will give you an idea of the information that we look at to determine your potential risk for Health issues including weight gain.

Candida will be covered in detail after we review some of the questions that are asked in the questionnaire.

The General Health Assessment (Candida Questionnaire)

In this section we're going to ask general questions about your health and wellbeing.

A sampling of the questions we would ask will include:

Do you feel tired most of the time?

Does the fatigue alter your lifestyle?

Do you have intestinal gas?

Do you crave sugar? Bread? Beer?

Do you have weight gain that's hard to lose?

Are you experiencing a loss of libido?

These are by no means all the questions, but they give you an example of the information we're looking for in this section of the assessment.

The Thyroid Assessment

On the next page of the assessment we'll talk about your thyroid function.

Do you have severe fatigue and find it hard to get up in the morning?

Do you have generalized low energy?

Do you need caffeine or other stimulants to get you going?

Do you have a family history of thyroid disease?

Do you gain weight easily?

Have you had difficulty losing weight in the last two years?

Do you have dry skin?

Again, this is a very classic thyroid function assessment. Many patients come in who have had normal thyroid blood tests but we know these don't always taken into account other factors, such as the basal body temperature and the functions of the thyroid, hypothyroidism, and not allowing for metabolism and healthy normalization of weight. The symptom assessment really helps to focus in on problems that blood tests can over look or not pick up.

The Stress Assessment

Are you happy with your current job, or profession?

Do you exercise regularly, three or more times per week?

Do you consume caffeine, sugar or refined carbohydrates?

Do you take down time to recharge your batteries?

Are you satisfied with your life and its direction?

Do you keep your weight within normal range easily?

Do you get eight hours of uninterrupted sleep per night?

Are you more tired after exercise?

This section is really focusing on and assessing the adrenal glands. When a person has adrenal stress the increase in cortisol, blood sugar and insulin in the body sends the body into a fat storing mode versus the fat burning mode we want to be in.

The Hormone Assessment

In this section the answers would be based on being male or female. We ask questions regarding hormones and whether they're in balance or if you're experiencing an imbalance. These questions are answered with a yes or no response.

Are you experiencing anxiety? Mood swings?
Sagging skin?
Poor sleep quality?
Memory problems?
Fatigue?
Hot flashes?
Salt and fluid retention?
Rapid weight gain?
Depression?
Infertility?

These are a few of the many questions that are asked to let us know if there is a hormone imbalance in the body. When there is a hormone imbalance in the body this can cause a lot of symptoms in the body, one of which is weight gain or difficulty losing weight.

The Toxic Burden Assessment

In this section we will ask questions about a person's diet. We want to know about your diet. We want to know what you're eating because a lot of people in America mistakenly think their diet is healthy because of the commercials they've seen on TV.
One of the first and most important questions of the toxic burden assessment is: How many fast food meals do you eat each week? The

answers range from none; one to two meals; or three or more meals per week. That one question is going to give us a lot of information on the toxins you're putting into your body. The more toxins you put in, the more acidic you are. The more acidic you are, the more weight you're going to gain.

Consider the following questions as well. They can generally be answered with a yes or no.

Do you consume diet foods sweetened with aspartame, splenda, saccharine?

Do you tend to overeat?

Do you consume damaged fats, hydrogenated oils or oxidized rancid fats? Fast foods fit into this area.

Do you regularly consume foods preserved with MSG?

Do you eat foods that are artificially colored?

Do you chew your food completely?

How many refined carbs or sugar servings do you eat per day?

Do you eat only organic produce grown with no pesticides?

How many different colors of vegetables and fruits do you eat each day?

Do you have an excessive consumption of soda, coffee; more than two cups or two cans a day?

These symptom assessments are going to help us to determine which program to put you on. This information is critical for our office and the doctors at Club Reduce®. It helps us determine and assess what program will work best for you

CANDIDA

In this section I want to talk about Candida, the yeast within. I have found while practicing and treating patients who are overweight have some Candida causing weight problems in both male and female.

As you look at the following questions keep track of how many you are answering yes to. When we're finished we'll help you rate whether Candida could be a problem for you.

1.   Do you feel tired most of the time?

2. Does the fatigue alter your lifestyle?

3. Do you suffer from intestinal gas?

4. Do you suffer with abdominal bloating or discomfort?

5. Do you crave vinegar, sugar, bread, beer or other alcoholic beverages?

6. Are you bothered by bowel disorder?

7. Are you bothered by Constipation? Diarrhea or alternating constipation and diarrhea?

8. Do you suffer from anxiety, depression, panic attacks or mood swings?

9. Are you often irritable, easily angered, anxious or nervous?

10. Do you have trouble thinking clearly or suffer memory loss, particularly short term memory loss?

11. Are you ever faint, dizzy or light headed?

12. Do you have muscle aches or take more than twenty four hours to recover from normal activities?

13. Without changes in your diet have you had weight gain and not been able to lose weight no matter what you have tried?

14. Does itching and burning of the vagina, rectum, and prostate bother you or have you experienced a loss of sexual desire?

15. Do you have a white or yellow fuzzy coating on your tongue?

16. Have you had athlete's foot, ringworm, jock itch or other chronic fungal infections of the skin or nails?

17. Does exposure to perfumes, insecticides, new carpeting or other chemical smells bother you?

18. Have you at any time in your life taken broad spectrum antibiotics? Tetracycline, Penicillin?

19. Are you using birth control or shots or have you ever used birth control or shots?

20. Are you on synthetic hormones?

21. Have you ever taken or had a steroid drug or had an injection for pain? These drugs are used for allergies, asthma, respiratory or injuries, cortisone, prednisone?

Now that you've answered these questions, you're going to rate your Candida probability.

If you answered yes to twelve or more of these questions you have a high likelihood of Candida.

If you answered yes to seven to eleven of these questions, you have a high probability of a Candida problem.

Five to six yeses indicate a moderate probability; and zero to four indicates a low probability, but you still may have some Candida.

Keep in mind, this self screening is provided for general information only and is not intended to be used for self diagnosis without the advice or examination of a health professional.

Candida is an over-infestation of yeast in the body. It invades the brain and every tissue of the body, much as the disease Fibroidmyalgia does. In a discussion about Fibroidmyalgia, it is important to address the condition of Candida as the symptoms of both conditions are exactly the same, with the exception of the touch points, or the hot tender spots of the back. The lifestyle change programs that these conditions require differ greatly.

Candida can be just as devastating as Fibroidmyalgia. However, unlike Fibroidmyalgia, Candida grows and lives on what you eat. It makes your body crave what it needs and it rampages until you give in to these cravings. For this reason Candida is difficult to get rid of but it can be eradicated if proper steps are taken.

Candida may occur alone or in combination with Fibroidmyalgia. About 80% of those suffering from Fibroidmyalgia also have Candida. Both of these syndromes are auto immune disorders. Take the touch point test to determine if your pain and fatigue may be caused by Fibroidmyalgia. This touch test on the back will determine how sensitive your muscles are.

If you suspect Fibroidmyalgia, you should also screen for Candida. We always screen for both syndromes before determining a program for the patients at our office. For our Candida screening test, take the self test below (shown previously). If your score leads you to believe that you may have Candida, request a full Candida test from a Club Reduce holistic practitioner.

Many people have either one condition or the other. For those with both Fibroidmyalgia and Candida, the Candida must be treated before the Fibroidmyalgia. Candida Albicans is one of the many different types of yeast. Yeast cells are able to grow on the surface of all living things and occur virtually everywhere. The fact is, we breathe, eat and drink them daily because they are part of our daily lives. We all have yeast growing in our skin, on other body surfaces and in our intestines. Normally our body's defense systems keep the total number of yeast cells under control, so Candida colonies in our intestinal tract are usually nothing to worry about.

Causes of Candida

There are over 900 species of yeast, but Candida Albicans is the major one found in the human body. In some ways it's very much like the yeast used in breads. Scientists are not sure why yeasts are in our bodies or what their exact functions are. The only thing we know for sure is they help decompose and recycle our bodies when we die. If they multiply too rapidly in our bodies they begin their job prematurely. That's why it's so important to keep the yeast in our bodies under control.

A number of conditions lead to Candida. These include: steroid drugs such as cortisone, birth control pills; and the use of antibiotics such as those used to control acne or various bacterial infections can invite the problem. Antibiotics can reduce the number of beneficial bacteria that normally help to keep the yeast under control. Antibiotics kill not only the bad but also the good bacteria in the body. Good or friendly bacteria work like a police force or army keeping the invading yeast from spreading through the body. As long as the body maintains a sufficient number of helpful bacteria to counter balance the effects of harmful bacteria, or yeast, the body remains healthy. Antibiotics kill the weakest link and then the next weakest. The strongest bacteria, like certain yeasts, survive and multiply. Antibiotics or a specific drug, cream or suppository are used to treat the symptoms, the yeast and bacteria left become stronger. We have created new strains and generations of mutant and very difficult to eradicate viruses, bacteria and yeast.

In reaction to this problem, the drug companies then create stronger and stronger antibiotics and anti-fungal to kill the stronger mutant yeast and bacteria. The more chemical stuffers for symptoms that a person uses, the harder it is and the longer it takes for the body to naturally eradicate the Candida. Microbial resistance to antibiotics has become a major health crisis. Antibiotic drugs also suppress immune cell production and diminish the strength of the immune system as a whole.

Poor nutrition and a sluggish or impaired immune system weakens the body's ability to fight off yeast; and stress and environmental pollutants can also play a role in reducing the body's control over Candida. When this happens, the yeast colonies grow rapidly and Candida results. Alcohol, caffeine, stress, and aging all destroy friendly bacteria in the system.

Sugar, gluten and meat encourage harmful bacteria in the intestines and can increase the growth of Candida.

One of the reasons people get acne is because there is an overabundance of yeast in the body. The yeast is also known as Candida. Candida is an over infestation of yeast in the body. It invades the brain and every tissue of the body. Candida grows and lives on what you eat and makes your body crave what it needs to survive. For this reason, Candida is difficult to get rid of but it can be eradicated if proper steps are taken.

EFFECTS OF CANDIDA

When yeast is in an overabundance there may be local yeast infection in the mouth, which is called thrush; in the gastrointestinal tract, causing gas; in the vagina, causing vaginal yeast infection; in the urinary tract causing bladder or kidney infection; in the prostate gland causing prostate troubles; on the skin causing hives and rashes; in the fingernail or toenail causing fungus of the nail bed.

Too much yeast can cripple the immune system causing chronic viral and bacterial infections or allergies. Yeast can damage the intestinal wall allowing food particles and toxins to enter the blood stream. The body then produces antibodies to fight these foreign substances and typical allergic reactions may occur such as eczema, hay fever, along with headaches, dizziness, heart palpitations, anxiety, fatigue and muscle aches.

There may be changes in the cells that contribute to the Candida condition. Yeast by-products or exhaust are two very toxic substances. Two toxins, Ethanol and acetaldehyde, in turn alter the ability of our cells in the following ways:

Red blood cells have difficulty passing into small capillaries. This can cause fatigue, dizziness, muscle aches or headaches.

White blood cells have trouble enveloping bacteria and foreign material and the body has trouble fighting infection.

Sugar has difficulty passing through cells. Insulin cannot do its job properly, causing low blood sugar and often weight gain.

Thyroid hormones have trouble passing through cells which causes the metabolism to slow down, often causing low body temperature, cold hand and feet, fatigue and intolerance to cold.

Minerals have trouble passing through cell walls causing fluid retention and electrolyte imbalance.

Messages passing from one cell to another have difficulty, causing muscle and nerve problems.

Enzymes are destroyed. Remember, enzymes are the chemical helpers in the body that help to build, break down and produce energy and heat. Yeast toxins can inactivate or destroy some of the enzymes and can result in slowing all of the functions of the body.

For example, enzymes help break down sugar stores to keep the blood sugar at ideal levels. When yeast overgrowth destroys enzymes, abnormally high or low blood sugar levels may develop.

SYMPTOMS OF CANDIDA

As we discuss these symptoms count and highlight how many of these symptoms you have currently or you have had in the last ten years.

*Allergic reactions such as congested nose
*Hives
*Dizziness, weakness
*Cramps, arthritis
*Depression
*Increased sensitivity to foods or chemicals
*Gastrointestinal problems--gas, bloating, abdominal pain, gastritis, gastric ulcer, heartburn, diarrhea, constipation, spastic colon
*Respiratory problems--frequent sore throat, mouth or canker sores, sinus infection, bronchial infection, chronic cough, asthma

*Cardiovascular problems--palpitations, rapid pulse rate. Candida does not directly affect the heart, but rather the hormones regulating cardiovascular system.

*Genital/urinary problems--yeast infections, itching or burning in the vagina or prostate. Urinary burning, frequent urination, lack of bladder control, bed wetting, menstrual cramping, PMS.

*Musculoskeletal problems-muscle weakness, night leg pain, muscle stiffness, especially neck and shoulder, slow reaction time, poor coordination, poor motor skills, falling, tendency to drop things. Yeast impairs the cells from receiving nutrients and eliminating waste and also affects the nerve muscle sending patterns.

*Skin infection--usually rash type in nature, typically under the breast, in the groin area or diaper area, diaper rash, hives.

*Central nervous system problems--headaches, sinus headaches, tension headaches, migraines, low blood sugar headaches, rapid blood sugar changes. High levels of stress hormones can cause anxiety, irritability, moodiness, restlessness, panic attacks, sudden anger, sleep disturbances, poor short term memory, inability to concentrate, fuzzy thinking and confusion; and fatigue, which may be caused by impaired metabolism and impaired enzyme production.

*One of the main symptoms is weight gain which results from an overgrowth of yeast and causes cravings for sugar, interferes with normal hunger, causes high insulin levels, low metabolism, low energy levels, and fatigue.

I've had patients who have had anywhere from ten to thirty five of these symptoms, and never knew they had a Candida problem. By eliminating the Candida, the people I've put on programs, depending on how much weight they want to lose, have phenomenal results; not to mention having the symptoms we just reviewed disappear completely.

When you come to our office we'll test you to determine if Candida is something that is plaguing you and preventing you from reaching the goal of your desired weight, energy level or sleeping habits, or anything that may be bothering you physically.

The Effects of Drug Intervention on Candida

In conventional medicine, often what happens is that a patient will finish a course of antibiotics or steroid drug and shortly end up with a yeast infection. Drugs that specifically address the fungus, or Candida, destroy some of the yeast. The yeasts that are not affected by the drug begin to colonize in vast numbers and become more and more drug resistant. As the yeast multiplies into its stronger state, they produce toxins that attack the body's defense and immune system. These same drugs used to treat the yeast infection also destroy the friendly bacteria or flora in the body that we need to function properly. As a result, there is no defense against the new, stronger fungus.

There are many drugs now being used to treat Candida. Without fail, these drugs produce a stronger strain of bacteria that invades the body after the drug is ended. They all have an overall high incidence of drug related adverse effects. In clinical response, up to 26% of patients have adverse reactions to these medications in addition to producing stronger strains of yeast. Most Candida symptom drugs are prescribed for ten weeks to two years. Below is a list of some of these medications and the side effects experienced while taking them.

Diflucan antifungal: The most common adverse events include headache, nausea, abdominal pain, vomiting and diarrhea. Warnings on this drug include overall incidents of drug related adverse events is 26%. There are high incidents of clinically significant hypoglycemia. Mothers treated for three or more months with 400-800 mg Diflucan per day have had infants with multiple congenital abnormalities. Diflucan is secreted in human milk and should not be taken by nursing mothers.

Sporanox: This is a synthetic antifungal used for the treatment of fungal infections in immune compromised and non immune compromised patients. Most common adverse events include nausea, rashes, vomiting, diarrhea, edema, fatigue and fever. The warnings include Sporanox should not be used for pregnant patients or women contemplating pregnancy.

Nystatin: Whose brand names are mycostatin, nilstat, nadostein, nystex, and nystop antifungal? The most common adverse events in the oral form of the medication are nausea, upset stomach, and diarrhea. Adverse events from the vaginal form are irritation.

Fungizone: This antifungal, polyene antibiotic for use with oral Candida. Used as a mouthwash for thrush. Most common adverse events include rash, gastrointestinal problems, nausea, vomiting and diarrhea.

Again, when a Candida stuffer is prescribed—(a symptom stuffing drug such as an antibiotic, a steroid of any kind, an antifungal)--the weakest yeast is eradicated. However, the remaining yeast mutates and the strongest survives. For the next outbreak, conventional medicine will prescribe higher and higher doses of antifungal. These make the yeast stronger and further weakens the immune system. Treating Candida with drugs stops the immediate discomfort but causes the yeast to come back with more strength; and more symptoms develop almost immediately upon the end of the drug intervention.

A HOLISTIC APPROACH
THE Solutions4 FIVE WEEK
OR TWELVE WEEK CANDIDA PROGRAM

Since Candida and other yeasts are all around us, we can never totally get rid of them. We can bring them back under control without the use of prescription drugs. To achieve the greatest degree of success an effective balance of dietary changes, nutritional support and the increase of friendly bacteria are necessary.

The Solutions4 detoxification and nutritional program will help provide this balance while teaching you how to keep yeast under control for good. There are some specific protocols for a Candida program which include detoxification; increasing the friendly bacteria; the use other supplements such as evening primrose oil and the Solutions4 multi vitamin and multi minerals; water; exercise; and a yeast control diet; plus all the other nutrients recommended for a yeast controlled Candida elimination program.

Detoxification, as in the case with any lifestyle change, involves a total cleanse of the system. This is the first step to improved health. Detoxification, as we mentioned in Chapter 3, along with a five week Candida nutritional program helps provide nutritional support to strengthen the immune system. A fully functional immune system and a diet that controls the intake of yeast will help reduce the Candida to a nonthreatening, harmless level. For those with both Candida and Fibroidmyalgia, treatment for Candida must occur before Fibroidmyalgia can be addressed successfully. Following the Candida program, we also have a Fibroidmyalgia program available for those with that condition.

In order to start to get well, the first step is to cleanse the body through detoxification. This is a total body cleansing program which cleanses the liver, bowels, kidneys and the blood supply. It helps restore the peristaltic action of the colon. It helps to rid the body of mucus, toxins and waste materials that are trapped in the colon and may have been there for years. Detoxification will help to rid your body of this condition for life. For specific instructions on the cleanse, again refer to Chapter 3.

Healing Crisis

As you're on the Candida program you may experience, at any time, a healing crisis. The healing crisis journey lasts from a few hours to a few days. The healthier one's body is when starting a program the fewer symptoms of healing crisis there will be. The more the body has to clean up, the harder and longer the cleansing side effects will be. The symptoms will also be more pronounced if the change in the diet is abrupt and less so if it is gradual. Live yeast will revolt in an aggravation of all symptoms. Things seem to get worse before they get better. We have patients call the office and tell us they're experiencing the symptoms of a healing crisis. This is perfect. That means your body is working exactly the way it should be and this is to be expected. All of the following are normal reactions to the cleansing process: stomach cramping, low grade fever during the days of detoxification, an orange discharge from the eliminative organs, and rapid weight loss after several days on the program. Candida will try to defeat you. Perseverance is the key. The more toxic you were the more healing crisis symptoms you will experience.

This is why detoxification preparation days are so important (see Chapter 3). Each healing crisis is followed by increased vitality and improved well-being. Please be aware that it is just as important for your body to come off detoxification correctly as it is to detoxify as it is to do the detox itself.

Your body is in a cleansing mode and will continue until clogging foods are reintroduced. As you finish detoxification continue taking your supplements and herbs until they are gone. Many of the ill feeling symptoms that you may have experienced will have already begun to disappear. In fact, the three to five day cleansing is pretty dramatic. You will have lost two to eight pounds and will have begun eliminating some of the five to twenty seven pounds of waste that are being stored in the colon. If you're on medication ask your prescribing doctor to work with you as you go through this program.

Slowly work your way back to foods after detoxification. Start consuming fresh fruit after day 22 of the program, due to the fact that fruit can feed Candida. Start including salads and vegetables. Some people choose to juice live foods for a few days before eating solid foods, allowing the body more time to heal and have greater energy and gain strength. Slowly work your way back to foods after detoxification. Your body is now clean and will no longer tolerate abuse. A couple of beers will make you drunk and you may become ill after eating pizza, or a candy bar. It may give you a headache.

All these foods are very unhealthy and your clean body is simply more sensitive to toxins. Contact your doctor or your local health care practitioner if you have any questions on healing crisis.
Nutrition is essential to health and wellness. 100% nutrition ensures that the organs of the body and the immune system are being strengthened while getting what they need to function at their full potential. For more information about food and nutrition refer again to Chapter 2.

THE YEAST CONTROLLING DIET

Following the detoxification process a yeast controlled diet will be prescribed to you. There are going to be some foods that we recommend you avoid totally and some foods that we recommend you add to your diet.

These foods are foods that we recommend you eliminate from your diet. Candida grows on all these foods. If you do eat any of these during the die-off period of your program, you may need to start the program over.

Foods to Avoid
Red meat and pork

All fruits fresh, canned or dried until yeast is abated after 22 days. Fresh lemon or lime juices may be used in water or as a substitute for vinegar in salad dressings and recipes.

All sugars and sugar containing food including table sugar, fructose, corn syrup, high fructose corn syrup, honey, molasses, maple sugar unless it's from the tree, the pure maple syrup, date sugar and rice syrups.

All white flour and white flour products.

All yeast containing pastries, bread, crackers, pastas, etc; including Brewer's yeast, B vitamins made from yeast, yeast breads, pastries, crackers and pretzels that contain yeast.

Alcoholic beverages

All fruit juices

Coffee and tea including herbal,

Old leftovers. If a food has been in the refrigerator for more than three days do not eat it. Leftovers may be frozen and consumed at a later date.

Obvious fungus foods, mushrooms, blue cheese.

All nuts. This is due to possible mold.

All processed meats such as bacon, sausage, ham, hot dogs, lunch and deli meats, corned beef and pastrami.

All vinegar soaked products or vinegar dressings, pickles, pickled relish, mustard, Tabasco sauce, etc. Lemon juice may be used as a substitute for vinegar in recipes.

Artificially sweetened drinks and food products. Avoid soft drinks.

Dairy products, milk, buttermilk, whipped cream, sour cream, ice cream. All cheese and dairy except butter and organic eggs, all hard cheeses are made from mold.

Corn and corn products, all grains including wheat, oats, barley, rye, sorghum, etc.

Implementing Friendly Bacteria

The human gastrointestinal tract is a home to many types and numbers of microbes or bacteria. Microbes live in our skin, in our mouths, in women's vaginal tracts, and throughout our gastrointestinal tract. It is estimated that there are more microbes, bacterial cells, than there are human cells in and on the human body. There is also a very large diversity of the types of bacteria with over 400 different species being present in humans. Because of the diversity in number, it has become evident that bacteria play an important role in human health. Most of these bacteria are not harmful and in fact contribute positively to normal growth and development. Some of these bacteria, however, can have negative influences. Keeping a healthy balance of the bacteria—(favoring beneficial bacteria over potentially harmful bacteria)--is essential to the proper functioning of all systems of the body. Friendly bacteria strains can suppress harmful bacteria. They have been shown to improve intestinal tract health by aiding digestion and elimination, alleviating the symptoms of lactose intolerance, improving absorption of minerals, reducing toxins in the blood stream and improving immune function.

Friendly bacteria are needed to manufacture and assimilate B vitamins, niacin, biotin, folic acid, riboflavin and B-12, produce digestive enzymes, detoxify toxic materials in the body, reduce unfriendly bacteria in the body, reduce blood pressure, reduce cholesterol in the blood, balance Ph levels in the intestines, the acid alkaline balance, assist in protection from colon irritation, constipation and diarrhea, helps with digestion of proteins, carbohydrates and fats, produce natural antibacterial agents, detoxify chemicals added to foods, increase assimilation of calcium, retard yeast growth (especially Candida), retard Candida infections, herpes; and helps eliminate bad breath, bloating, and gas.

What destroys natural friendly bacteria in the system? Again, as we discussed earlier, antibiotics kill not only the bad but also the good bacteria in the body. This includes the antibiotics in the meat and dairy products that we consume each day. Even one dose of these things can kill all the friendly bacteria. If you consume any foods at fast food restaurants for lunch or dinner those foods, you're consuming the antibiotics in that food. Steroid drugs, cortisone, birth control, laxatives, and alcohol destroy enzymes and the lacto bacteria. Coffee destroys friendly bacteria. Stress aging, anything that weakens the immune system, also affects the balance of beneficial and harmful bacteria.

What encourages harmful bacteria in the intestines? Sugar and any foods containing white sugar and sugar substitutes. Foods that contain gluten, bread and pastries are Candida producing. Meat feeds the bacillus coli its harmful bacteria which then overrun the friendly bacteria; and any foods that use fermentation or mold in the production process.

What are the effects of an unhealthy balance of bacteria? Some of the most common effects are diarrhea and digestive problems, lactose intolerant, hypertension, cancer, small bowel, bacterial overgrowth, kidney stones, elevated blood cholesterol and allergies. The Solutions4 Probiotic formula provides friendly bacteria and using this formula as part of the Solutions4 Candida program will help maintain a healthy level of friendly bacteria in the system to allow the body to keep yeast under control.

Water consumption. Water is critical to the treatment of any health condition including Candida. Every organ of the body requires water. The heart, lungs and skin and circulatory system all depend on water. To calculate your individual need divide your weight in half. Half of your body weight gives you a good rule of thumb for how many ounces of water your body needs to function on a daily basis. For example, if you weigh 150 pounds you must drink 75 ounces of water each day. Nothing substitutes for water. If you drink enough water each day you absolutely will feel different. This is not to say you can't drink other liquid, but remember the importance of the quantity of water that you drink each day. Have water in your car, house, and office; consume and drink water.

Evening Primrose oil is another product we'll discuss more in detail later. This is an important nutrient. The gamma linolenic acid, GLA, as well as linseed oil, is a rich source of linolenic acid. Recent research has shown that polyunsaturated fatty acids are needed by the body for building cells and for the production of prostaglandulan which controls many body functions including the immune system. These supplements help to ensure the body is receiving an adequate supply.

Exercise and fitness. Some of my patients have a hard time exercising because they have little motivation and when they do exercise they actually feel worse. If this is the case, you will want to begin a program of exercise gradually. Go at a comfortable pace. Start at five minutes a day and then work to ten and then to thirty minutes. Even though fatigue and muscle soreness is a symptom of Candida, exercise is vital. Do cardiovascular exercises, walking briskly, swimming, treadmill, stairs, biking, etc. Exercise at least three times per week working up to thirty minutes each time. Get plenty of fresh air and sunshine. Exercise is also an excellent antidepressant. Mental exercise is important. Set aside time daily to relax, unwind, de-stress and allow positive emotional and psychological repair to begin.

APPROVED FOODS FOR THE CANDIDA DIET

The amount of vegetables consumed on the Solutions4 program is unlimited. Use the list below for successful eating. Vegetables may be steamed for four minutes or stir fried over low heat, but for best results at least half of your vegetable intake should be raw. Vegetable intake should be twice the amount of fruit intake. Remember, fruits are only allowed after the first twenty two days of the program.
Use organic products when possible. Using frozen vegetables is okay, however, no dried or canned vegetables. Fresh juices made from vegetables are allowed. The standard serving size of vegetable juice is half a cup. Fresh herbs and spices may be used, but do not use any dried herbs or spices.

The Allowed Vegetables: artichokes, alfalfa sprouts, asparagus, avocado, bamboo shoots, bean sprouts, beets, bok Choy, broccoli, Brussels sprouts, buckwheat sprouts, Red and Chinese cabbage, carrots, cauliflower, celery, chard, chives, cucumber, eggplant, fennel, garlic, green beans, green onion, kohlrabi, lima beans, leek, mung bean sprouts, okra, olives, onion, parsley, parsnip, peas, pepper, green pepper, red pepper, pimento, radish, rhubarb, rutabaga, shallots, snap beans, edible pods, snow peas, sugar peas, string beans, sprouts, sunflower sprouts, tomatillos, tomatoes, turnips, water chestnut, wheat grass, zucchini, lettuce and greens, arugula, beet greens, Belgium endive, bib lettuce, Boston lettuce, butter lettuce, cress, collard greens, curly endive, dandelion greens, endive, red endive, escarole, green leaf iceberg, kale, mustard greens, oak leaf, radicchio, red leaf romaine, spinach, Swiss chard, and water cress.

The Allowed Fruits: After twenty two days you can add fruit back into your diet. Why can't I have fruit for the first 22 days on the program? One of the reasons you cannot have fruit for the first 22 days is because Candida lives on the fruit because of the sugar content of the natural sugar that's in the fruit. So we're trying to starve out the yeast. Once you have finished the first 22 days of the program, you may begin to include the following fruits into your diet: apples, apricots, bananas, blackberries, blueberries, boysenberry, cantaloupe, cherry, coconut (Raw), dates, figs, grapefruit, grape, guava, kiwi, honeydew, lemon, lime, mango, melon, mulberry, nectarine, oranges, papaya, peaches, pears, persimmon, pineapple, plum, pomegranate, raspberries, strawberries, tangelo, tangerine, watermelon. Slowly introduce the fruit back into the diet. You should only try one piece of fruit and watch for symptoms to make sure the Candida is gone? For some people it may take longer than 22 days.

The Allowed Meats: Meat can be eaten after the initial detoxification period, however, get as lean a cut of meat as possible. The standard serving size is three ounces cooked, two to four servings per day with one to two of those servings being fish. The approved meats include: organic poultry, (free range, antibiotic free and hormone free is best), chicken, turkey, duck, and quail. Organic fish wild caught and not farm raised, cod, halibut, mahi-mahi, salmon, sea bass, sol is okay, swordfish, tilapia, trout, or tuna. Organic rabbit is allowed. Canned fish.

Lentils and rice: For best results on the Candida program lentils are recommended over rice because of the higher protein content of lentils. Included lentils and rice are: brown lentils, red lentils, basmati rice, brown rice, wild rice.

Eggs and Diary: Organic eggs, two per week or unlimited organic Egg Beaters; organic butter, used sparingly; coconut milk, raw, taken from a baby Thai coconut. No packaged milk is allowed.

Oils: Coconut oil is a great substitute for butter; extra virgin olive oil; flaxseed oil is great for dressings, however keep refrigerated and do not heat flax oil; grape seed oil, using only cold pressed and unprocessed.

Salt and spices: Salt, red salt or Celtic sea salt, real salt. Any spice in its whole form. Mixed seasonings generally have sugar and other preservatives.

Juices: Juices, fresh vegetable juices, fresh fruit juices (but only after day twenty two).

Water: distilled water preferred only when detoxifying; then filtered water, pure water, spring water. Remember to drink half your body weight in ounces of water.

Solutions4 nutritional shake: You have the option to replace one meal per day with a meal shake. The Solutions4 shake has amino acids, vitamins, minerals, twenty grams of healthy protein. It also is non dairy and lactose free and will be covered more in the supplement section chapter.

Foods and Beverages to avoid

Avoid alcohol, caffeine, tobacco and other stimulants. Avoid coffee and tea (including herbal), all dairy, all hard cheese are made from mold except organic eggs and butter. All sugar and sugar containing foods, refined sugar, fructose, corn syrup, high fructose corn syrup, honey, cane sugar, molasses, date sugar, maple syrup. Maple sugar is allowed on detox days--; only maple syrup.

All white flour and white flour products, all yeast containing pastries, crackers, breads, pasta, all grains except brown rice and lentils.

Meat, beef, lamb, pork, veal, shellfish, no cured smoked luncheon meats, all nuts and seeds, anything processed or refined.
Refined white flour and white sugar.

MSG or chemicals.

Foods or condiments that contain vinegar, molds or aged foods.
Avoid starchy vegetables, hominy, white rice, yams, potatoes, corn, and dried beans.

Structuring your diet on the five week Candida program

When not detoxing, your diet should consist mostly of green leafy vegetables. The easiest way to incorporate more greens in your diet is to plan meals around salads. An easy way to get your daily amount of fruit after day 22 is to have it for breakfast in the morning or add it to the nutritional shake. Rice and lentils are allowed on the program, but use them sparingly. Add your rice or lentils to a green salad to get more greens in the meal.

Why should my diet consist mostly of raw green leafy vegetables? Foods that require cooking to be consumed probably are not good nutritionally for humans even before cooking. By cooking them we further compromise their nutritional value because the vitamins and minerals, enzymes, co-enzymes and carbohydrates, proteins and fats are damaged or destroyed by heat of cooking.

What we get with grains after they have been cooked is the maximum amount of calories within the amount of nutrients. Salads are central to a raw diet and should be used to structure your meals. Structure your diet by building every meal around salads.

Successful eating tips for Candida

* Remember everything you need to live can be found in the produce section.
* Shop two times a week in order to get fresh produce.
* Most leafy greens have a refrigerator shelf life of four to five days.
*Buy your produce first. It's the most important food. If you're on a budget, shopping for produce will maximize your dollar as you avoid junk food while you have a cart full of produce.
* Wash leafy greens by separating the leaves. Rinse well in order to remove pesticides.
* Keep your refrigerator well stocked with fresh vegetables. This way you will always have what you need for a delicious salad. While shopping, ask yourself "how will this go with a salad?" Try to consider everything as something that will go into a salad or alongside it.
* Take Solutions4 digestive enzyme blend supplements with every meal. That will help to digest and break down the food and give the energy needed.
* Eat a variety of foods in a rainbow of colors.
* If using salt, use real salt or sea salt.
* Eat five to six small meals throughout the day. It will keep your metabolism going.
* Eat the last meal of the day before 6:00 p.m.
* Track calories. Women should have 1000 to 1100 per day. Men should have 1200 to 1300 per day. When you're eating this much raw food and vegetables 1000 calories of this type of food is really a lot of food.
* Go to bed early and get at least eight hours of sleep.

LIVING WITH THE CANDIDA DIET

Living on a diet that controls Candida isn't always going to be easy. Our American diet has been primed to eat certain foods, convenience foods that are destroying our health. There will be foods out there that tempt you to eat, but the results are never worth the momentary satisfaction.

I remember a patient of ours who had been in the Candida program and had been successful. She had been married for forty years and wanted to go out for a celebration. I recommended for her some raw food restaurants in our city. Her husband, however, really wanted to eat Chinese food, so she went along to the Chinese restaurant and ate. She called me the next day and explained to me how sick she was from the foods she ate there. I saw her two days later and she said that was the sickest she had been in years. In a sense, this is a good thing. In the past, when she was unhealthy, she could eat those foods and have no reaction to them. Because she was now healthy, her body was rejecting those foods and responding negatively to the toxic barrage of chemically processed MSG laden foods she had consumed.

We certainly don't recommend that you never go out to eat or go on vacation. When you do, try to eat as close to Candida friendly as possible. If you go on a three day trip, for example, when you come home begin preparation for a detox. Take your two preparation days eating no meats, no dairy and no grains. The next three days complete the lemonade detoxification program. If you went on a five day trip, try to do the lemonade detox for five days. By the end of this time period you will have cleansed the body from your trip and can continue on with your Candida friendly diet.

Another success story I'd like to share with you involves a 44 year old female patient that came in. After she filled out her assessment and had been screened we discovered she had high levels of Candida--up to 60.61%. Following her five week program she went down to 13%. All the areas of her assessment improved. Here is her story in her words: "I feel incredible and it's been years since I felt so good. My body feels like it's functioning properly and in balance. While doing my program I was pleasantly surprised at the increase in my energy levels, even while detoxifying. I am very pleased with my results. I have lost weight, inches and I think my appearance just looks healthier. My coworkers and family have noticed and complimented and congratulated me. Before I did this program my favorite foods were sweets, breads, dairy; and now my cravings for these are gone. My eating and cooking habits have changed and my family is benefitting from it. They are more aware of the foods they choose to eat. I sleep great. I have more energy for exercise and my busy lifestyle, my mood swings are minimal. I have better focus and concentration skills, no more foot odor and most of all I am happier. The list goes on and on and to think it's all due to a major diet change. Is this Amazing or is the body amazing to be able to heal itself if feed the proper foods. It wasn't easy but it was worth it."

Stories like these are what I see every day in my office, from patients that have come in with a Candida condition. As they cleanse, as they detoxify their bodies and heal we have patient after patient, story after story, people changing their lives. Their lives are not only changing and improving, but the lives of their families are as well. For example, children who eat this way they do better in school. Husbands and wives who eat this way are able to lose weight and keep the Libido going strong for years. It's just an amazing program.

As you come into the office and get tested with this symptom assessment form we can determine if you have Candida present in your body. Again, Candida programs will be determined once you come into the office and fill out the symptom assessment. The Candida program will be explained to you and the length of the program will determine how much weight you'd like to lose. Your program will include all the supplements you need and the products that we'll be describing in the Supplement chapter. We will give you guidelines, recipes, and menu plans. We will explain to you what you need to do, and how everything works. The detoxification and cleansing process will be explained to you in the office.

Our office has proudly helped thousands and thousands of patients with amazing results. This program works 100% of the time; and so I am very pleased and happy with the way we've been able to help people gain improved health then loose the weight. We have doctors all across the country doing the same program; so if you need to find a doctor in your specific area, go to www.Solutions4.com and find a doctor near you using the provider locater tab.

CHAPTER
FIVE

Hormones – Thyroid, Adrenals

CHAPTER FIVE
HORMONES

What are hormones?

Hormones are chemical messengers which are produced and secreted by numerous glands in the body. Once a hormone is released into the blood stream as a result of a certain stimuli, it instructs target cells and/or glands to produce a particular substance such as other hormones. These hormones stimulate or inhibit the actions of cells everywhere, depending on the needs of the body. Thus, although very different in their functions, different hormones are dependent on each other to produce a balanced chemical environment in the body. For example, glands such as the ovaries, adrenals, pituitary and hypothalamus produce and regulate levels of estrogen, progesterone, and androgens.

Estrogen

What is estrogen for? What does it do? Estrogen causes the growth of sexual organs, causes the lining of the uterus to thicken and endometrial glands to develop and nourish a fertilized egg. It causes an increase in overall body fat which gives soft, fine-textured skin. It causes fluid and salt retention in the tissues to plump and fill skin. It helps retain calcium in the bones and has a direct effect on the endothelial lining of blood vessels; affects physiological functions of the body like blood sugar, emotional balance and memory. It has stimulatory effects on the nervous system. High levels can trigger anxiety, irritability and mood swings. It is used by the body for cellular growth and repair; and it inhibits the osteoclast, the cells that tear down old bone. It can cause weight gain and hot flashes when a shortage occurs. The symptoms of menopause result mainly from a progesterone deficiency relative to estrogen. It's an anti-libido hormone.

A brief history of Hormone Replacement Therapy, HRT

HRT, or hormone replacement therapy, came of age in the late 1960s, although it had been studied as early as the 1930s, according to

Sherill Sellman in her book Hormone Heresy. The early research using hormones and organs from monkeys showed little effectiveness and even resulted in dire consequences. But in 1966, after years of refocusing research on synthetic estrogen instead of animal derived products, the pharmaceutical companies emerged triumphant, changing the medical landscape and women's bodies forever.

In 1966 Dr. Robert Wilson, a New York gynecologist, wrote a bestseller called Feminine Forever. His message was that estrogen replacement would save women from the tragedy of menopause, which often destroys her character as well as her health. The book, it turns out, was paid for by pharmaceutical giant Wyeth-Ayerst. The author's foundation, the Wilson Research Foundation also was financed by Wyeth, along with other drug companies that had interest in creating a market for their new drugs.

Thanks to Wilson's book and lectures, Wyeth's estrogen replacement drug became the fifth leading prescription drug in the US by 1975, just about the time researchers found that such drugs could increase the risk of uterine cancer at remarkable rates. The solution? Don't stop the estrogen. Just add progesterone. Progesterone seemed to counter the effects of estrogen on the uterine lining, making the wonder cure for women safe again--for a while.

Hormone replacement therapy marketing

The media has become a huge tool for pharmaceutical companies. This has progressed over time to the point where you can't watch television without seeing all the clever advertising that's being done. Instead of allowing the doctors to make recommendations on if or when pharmaceuticals are needed, the general public is going to their doctors telling them what drugs they should be on--simply because they saw the ad on television extolling the benefits. The media is garnering record advertising dollars from pharmaceutical companies; a trend that's not changing any time soon.

PMS and Menopause become Diseases

In mainstream medicine hormonal symptoms, PMS and menopause, are seen as hormonal deficiencies for which routine treatment is synthetic hormone replacement. The conventional medical approach is to force a woman's body to live with a hormone level associated with childbearing years. This doesn't take into account that the healthy human body has organs that produce and balance hormones naturally if given the proper environment.

Hormones and Aging

Hormones direct our bodies telling us when to grow, when to slow and every step to take in between. Hormone levels change over a lifetime, presenting special challenges in transitional periods. This is particularly true for women experiencing menopause. The amount of estrogen produced by the ovaries affect the length and timing and even the amount of flow in a woman's menstrual cycle. As ovaries age, they may not release an egg every month. When this happens estrogen causes the uterine lining to continue to build. Thus, a thicker lining results in a heavier flow. A woman's cycle may come closer together and she may experience gushing as well as notice a thicker flow than usual.

Eventually, ovaries will produce less estrogen and a cycle's flow will become lighter because there is less to shed. When ovaries no longer produce estrogen, a woman will skip a cycle altogether or stop having periods completely. This is known as menopause, the physical transition in which women lose the ability to reproduce.

The US population is aging. The subgroup within this aging population, which is growing at the greatest rate, is post-menopausal women. The average age of menopause, age 52, hasn't changed since 1950; however female life expectancy has greatly increased. Females in 1850 often did not live long enough to reach menopause, at a life expectancy of only 47 years. Today women are living into their 80s which means one third of their lives are being spent being post menopausal and menopausal.

Pre-menopause and menopause are natural hormone transitional periods in the human life cycle, much like that of puberty and should be experienced as a natural stage of life, not treated like a disease. The prevailing myth in mainstream medicine is that menopause is an estrogen deficiency disease. Although estrogen levels do decrease at menopause, they drop only 40-60% while progesterone levels can drop as well.

The FDA's Stand on HRT

According to WebMD January 8th 2003, the US Food and Drug Administration, the FDA, has asked that all labels on estrogen and estrogen progestin replacement therapy be revised to carry a boxed warning stating the increased risk for heart disease, heart attack, stroke and breast cancer. The warning also emphasizes that these products are not approved for heart disease prevention.

"We have approved all new labeling for WYETH Pharmaceuticals for Prempro, Premarin, and Premphase", said the FDA spokesperson Pam Winbourne in a teleconference with reporters. "All other manufacturers are being faxed letters asking them to revise their labels in a similar fashion. We believe that different estrogens and progestin act similarly and in absence of data otherwise, women need to assume the risk with other estrogens and progestin's are similar", said Ms Winbourne. Other studies do show that estrogen and progestin are associated with these same side effects. The label also urges that physicians prescribe the lowest dose of estrogen and estrogen progestin products and for the shortest duration to achieve treatment goals.

The label changes reflect findings from the Women's Health Initiative, WHI, a landmark study that found overall health risks for estrogen and progestin, particularly for invasive breast cancer, heart attacks, blood clots; and that these risks exceed benefits of fractures and colon cancer risk reduction said Ms. Winbourne.

The FDA also conducted its own review of data from the WHI and confirmed the study's findings. "We are assuming that labels have accurate information as uncovered by the WHI", she said. "The black box warning asks that decisions about using hormone replacement therapy balance the benefits and potential risks. Our actions also include new guidance for conduct of clinical trials developing products for vaso-motor symptoms and vulvar and vaginal atrophy," Ms. Winbourne added, "including treatments of the following symptomatic conditions: moderate to severe vaso-motor symptoms, hot flashes and night sweats. The FDA still believes that these products are highly effective and very valuable in treating moderate to severe symptoms of hot flashes and night sweats said Ms. Winbourne.

These symptoms can be very disruptive and can often only be controlled by estrogen products. That will not change."
Vaginal and vulvar atrophy, the new label states that when estrogen products are being considered only for the conditions of vaginal and vulvar atrophy, topical vaginal products should be considered. In the prevention of osteoporosis, the new label states that when prescribing solely for this condition estrogen should only be considered for women at significant risk for osteoporosis and that non estrogen treatment such as bi-phosphonates should be carefully considered. Some 6.5 million women in the US now take some form of hormone replacement therapy, HRT, Winbourne said.

Estrogens added to list of Carcinogens--USA Today, January 6th 2003.

The federal government has added estrogens used in post-menopausal hormone therapy and oral contraceptives to its official list of known human carcinogens. An advisory panel of the National Institute of Environmental Health Science ruled that steroidal estrogen should be listed because of an association with endometrial cancer; and to a lesser extent, breast cancer.

The number of substances deemed known or reasonably accepted to pose a cancer risk stands at 228. The report doesn't address potential benefits of the product. It does note that birth control pills containing estrogen might protect against ovarian cancer.
Estrogen warning urged, February 23rd 1994

Researchers, citing the growing link between environmental estrogen and breast cancer, say prevention is needed. HRT interferes with metabolism of natural estrogen. Dr. Elihu Richter, from Hebrew University, told the American Association for the Advancement of Science that woman aged sixty to sixty six on estrogen replacement therapy have an 87% increased breast cancer risk.

ERT, estrogen replacement therapy, cuts the risk of heart disease and osteoporosis but has the highest cancer risks. "Should breast cancer be the price we pay for reduced risk of heart disease and fractures?" asks Dr. Graham Colditz, of Harvard Medical School. His answer was no.

Rethinking Hormone Therapy

The following is from Dr. Andrew Weils, Self Healing, September 2002:. Millions of women who take the hormone estrogen and progestin were recently thrown for a loop when results from the first large clinical study of hormone replacement therapy, HRT, were released. The findings from the Women's Health Initiative, WHI, show that long term use of HRT not only didn't reduce the risk of heart disease as previously thought, but actually increased a woman's risk of developing cardiovascular problems and breast cancer.

The WHI study followed some 16,000 women ages fifty to seventy nine who took either a combination of estrogen and progestin or a placebo pill. Although the eight year study was supposed to last until 2005, it was stopped when researchers determined that the risks of taking HRT outweighed the benefits. In fact, it was found that women taking HRT were more likely to develop invasive breast cancer or suffer a stroke, heart attack or blood clot than women not taking the hormones. The increased risk of breast cancer became evident after about four years of HRT use, but the cardiovascular risk appeared just a year or two on the drugs. Women taking HRT did appear to have reduced risk of colo-rectal cancer and hip fractures - Journal of American Medical Association, July 17th 2002.

What happened? The National Institute of Health, sponsor of the WHI, suddenly pulled the plug three years early on the study seeking to determine whether hormone replacement therapy could prevent major chronic illness. For years we as women have been told that staying on synthetic hormones during the imbalance years of our lives would make us younger and keep us healthy. Because of the statistically significant number of women in the study getting breast cancer, researchers concluded that it was unethical to continue.

The research provided other alarming findings. There was a 41% increase in strokes, 29% increase in heart attacks, doubling rate of blood clots, 22% increase in total cardiovascular disease, 26% increase in breast cancer. These findings contradicted almost all medical predictions and essentially called into question previous studies done on HRT. Upon stopping the trial the federal government immediately sent a letter to 16,000 participants and their doctors advising them to stop taking the drugs.

In an editorial accompanying the study, Dr. Susan Fletcher and Dr. Graham Coldiz of Harvard Medical School said the whole purpose of healthy women taking long term estrogen progestin therapy is to preserve health and prevent disease. The results of this study provide strong evidence that the opposite is happening for important aspects of women's health, even if the risk is low. Given these results we recommend that clinicians stop prescribing for long term use. The study found that risks clearly outweigh benefit.

Hormone therapy was also believed to prevent fractures due to osteoporosis, but the new study raises questions about that too. Women in the trial who were on hormones had a slightly higher rate of hip fractures than those taking the placebo, the opposite of what was expected.

The media has portrayed these results as a bombshell, but I'm not surprised. For years I have warned women about the increased risk of breast cancer from HRT, because exposure to estrogen stimulates the proliferation of breast tissue; and while many physicians have recommended that some women take HRT in order to prevent cardiovascular problems, this theory has never been proved in a randomized, controlled study like the WHI.

Also, the WHI study used a popular but unnatural hormone drug called Prempro which combines Premarin and estrogen obtained from the urine of pregnant horses with synthetic progesterone called progestin. Although the doses used in the study reflect those used by most women on HRT, other research suggests that those doses are higher than what may be needed to mitigate menopausal symptoms. More research needs to be done but I suspect that lower doses of bio-identical versions of estrogen and progestin are the same as those made naturally by the human body, maybe safer.

Bio-identical hormones are also new on the horizon and have been used for several years. Some experts have claimed that they have the same results as HRT, the same risk, but there haven't been any follow up studies for these bio-identical hormones yet.

So what's a woman to do? There is no single right answer. Deciding when and if to do HRT and what forms to use are individual decisions that each woman needs to discuss with her doctor. HRT is quite effective at managing hot flashes and other menopausal symptoms, but many women can cope with these effects through natural approaches alone. We have had a lot of success in helping women with these hormonal imbalances with natural hormone pre-cursers that give the body the ingredients to make hormones natural and when needed.

I would advise against taking HRT to prevent heart disease given this new evidence as taken from Dr. Weils and consider all options.

Hormone Health

Hormone health does not depend on using toxic doses of synthetic drugs to suppress symptoms. Like any aspect of health, hormone health is linked directly to having essential 100% nutrition, exercise, stress control and detoxification to produce and metabolize hormones properly. Given the proper environment, the body is able to manufacture its own balanced hormones.

As we go back in women's history before the 1960s, the environment we were exposed to on a daily basis was not as toxic as it is today. In 1996 researchers had identified at least 51 synthetic chemicals that disrupt the hormonal balance system. These toxins cause gonadal, thyroid, pituitary, and adrenal dysfunction, which compromise the immune system, hormone production and homeostasis. These toxins can also cause developmental defects in cellular reproduction such as breast cancer.

Human mad, or synthetic, hormones mimic natural hormones. However they are not bio-identical to naturally made hormones. The body can break down and excrete natural plant precursors, compounds, and use them to balance hormone health. Synthetic hormones are toxic and do not eliminate from the body.

Hormone drugs are consumed in animal foods--meat, beef, poultry, and pork. These animal proteins have been injected with growth hormones and antibiotics. Milk or milk products in which the cows have been given growth hormone, or any other animal food source, may contain hormones which alter the body's hormone balance. There is an alarming example of what is happening to our culture by the addition of synthetic hormones in our food supply. This is the trend of seven and eight year old girls beginning their menstrual cycles in the third and fourth grades, rather than at the age of twelve to fourteen as has historically been the case.

Symptoms of Improper Hormone Balance

In preteens and teens: menstrual cramping, bloating, acne, mood swings, heavy blood flow.

In the childbearing years, 20s and 30s: PMS, migraines, infertility, bloating, weight gain. Excess body fat is a risk factor for heart disease, high blood pressure, diabetes, breast cancer and stroke.

Weight gain in the 30s and 40s is very common in both men and women. Changes in hormone levels during the aging process aid in the distribution and storage of body fat in and near your midsection. Postpartum depression and tender breasts are also common.

In perimenopause, the transition period when hormone levels decrease, the menstrual cycle is erratic. This can last up to ten years. Other symptoms include loss of sex drive, hair loss, mood swings, weight gain, bloating, night sweats, acne, sleep deprivation, depression, bone loss, cancer, and hot flashes.

Menopause is the permanent cessation of menstruation with at least one year without menstrual cycle. The symptoms are hot flashes, osteoporosis, depression, Alzheimer's and heart disease.

During post menopause these symptoms gradually decline.

Does What I Eat Matter?

In the inception of Solutions4, the beneficial international company, Dr. Linda Nelson launched spas in Asia and began exploring the health and wellness aspects that would form the basis for our products and programs. What she discovered was the lack of menopause and menstrual symptoms that are so common in Western cultures was amazing. Studies show that the diet in Asian cultures is high in plant sterols. Plant sterols are easily converted to human estrogen and progesterone by the body. As a result, Asian women rarely experience the symptoms that Western cultured women consider biologically normal.

The difference between getting hormones from pills and animal products that have been fed synthetic hormones and those from plants is that in plant form you are simply ingesting precursors. Your body utilizes and converts only what it needs, allowing for natural and healthy hormone levels.

Foods that supply plant hormone precursors include soy, flax seed, yams, peas, cucumbers, bee pollen, raw nuts, seeds, papaya, banana, licorice root, raw fruits, juices of raw fruits and vegetables, leafy greens, garlic, avocado, grapes, apples, wheat germ, wheat grass and cherries. When introducing foods that are estrogen and progesterone precursors, the body doesn't replace lost hormones with synthetic, but instead stimulates the body to correct its own hormone imbalance. In the case of menopausal symptoms it is an imbalance, not a shortage that actually produces the symptoms. The body is trying to return to its natural state.

Natural Progesterone

Synthetic progestin is chemically formulated from natural progesterone, but they are not its chemical equivalent. Your body can normally convert a hormone into other hormones when needed. Synthetics cannot be converted by the body and they also produce many side effects. Natural progesterone and precursors are considered bio-identical, meaning chemically identical to those naturally produced by the body. When these two are combined, they are converted by the adrenal gland into corticosteroids and aldosterone, endrogen, estrogen, cortisol, DHEA, pregnenolone and adrenaline.

Functions of Progesterone:

*   Stimulates secretory activity in the body
*   Acts as a sedative with a calming effect
*   Normalizes blood sugar levels
*   Pressures all other steroid hormones including estrogen and cortisol

* Causes regression of tumors induced by estrogen
* Stimulates osteoblasts, the cells that make new bone formation
* Regulates metabolism, making it more efficient, utilization of fat for energy
* Opposes the effects of stress
* Causes weight loss by improving the body's efficiency in burning fuel for energy and eliminating fluids.
* Is a natural diuretic
* Prevents stress induced coronary
* Is linked to delayed aging and longer life span
* Balances estrogen to relieve hot flashes
* Is a pro libido hormone
* Protects against cancer
* Enhances thyroid hormone
* Increases antidepressant activity
* Blocks estrogen side effects

Androgens, the Male Testosterone Hormone
* Maintains sex drive
* Maintains muscle strength
* Maintains lean muscle mass
* Maintains body weight
* Regulates hair growth

As the body goes through the progression of disease the immune system breaks down and hormone imbalance almost always comes into play. Symptoms are always a late manifestation of a breakdown in the body. The breakdown generally occurs long before symptoms surface. 95% of all degenerative disease begins with a toxic colon. Thus, it makes sense that to achieve hormone balance you must first target the source in the body by detoxifying the body as discussed in Chapter Three.

Creating and maintaining hormone balance requires detoxifying the body, reducing caffeine and alcohol intake, practicing stress management techniques, taking the proper supplements to rebuild the immune system, and eating a natural precursor diet.

Years ago we used to be able to go to the zoo and feed the animals; but eventually the animals started to get sick and die from the junk and processed foods people fed them. Now the zoo has signs that say "Do not feed the animals". According to the World Health Organization processed foods are the cause of increased obesity levels and disease including cancer and heart disease. Processed foods with all the nutrients taken out aren't good for humans and they aren't good for animals either.

Humans can also get sick and die from eating junk food, yet our society continues to send out messages that it's okay to eat junk and fast food. These messages come from a multibillion dollar industry. We are constantly bombarded with advertising that promotes obesity and poor health. The advertising is not going away. Therefore, you must take responsibility for yourself to learn how to be healthy so you can lose weight and start living; start by educating yourself and your family.

Back in the 1950s, there was an ad for a Cola drink. The ad was promoting this cola as something good and healthy. The ad read this way: "Laboratory tests over the last few years have proven that babies who start drinking soda during that early formative period have a much higher chance of gaining acceptance and fitting in during those awkward preteen and teen years. So do yourself a favor. Do your child a favor. Start them on a strict regimen of sodas and other sugary carbonated beverages now for a lifetime of guaranteed happiness--promotes active lifestyle, boosts personality, gives the body essential sugars."

We might think that's crazy but these kinds of ads are still out there. On a bag of potato chips it says: "Happiness is Simple: It takes twelve muscles to smile, or three simple ingredients." How about this? If your child is upset, buy him a Happy Meal. Make him happy. All these toxins from our diets increase the risk of breast cancer, thyroid, pituitary gonadal dysfunction as well as developmental defects in cellular reproduction.

The problem gets worse every year because as Sally gets busier and busier in her fast paced lifestyle she eats fast foods and prepackaged foods from a box, bag or can to save time. Sally's body is not getting the nutrients it needs. She's starving so her body holds on to more and more fat. Nutrition plays a vital role in balancing hormones.

Cleanse and Clean:
Healthy Eating to Help Balance Hormones

It's important to try to eat organically-grown produce and also meats without steroids when trying to balance hormones. There are additional supplements that can be taken to help balance hormones. The following are symptoms of hormone imbalance. Note that these symptoms may also indicate the presence of Candida that we discussed in Chapter Four, the overgrowth of yeast in the body.

*Depression
*Mood swings,
*Violence
*Self Injury
*Drug Excesses
*Circles under the eyes
*Stiffness
*Eye Irritation, eye puffiness
*Cold extremities
*Constipation
*Tender breasts
*Greasy hair
*Fainting
*Migraines
*Epilepsy
*Frustration
*Joint pain
*Muscle pain
*Lethargy
*Asthma
*Runny nose, sore throat
*Herpes
*Headaches
*Aggression
*Irritability
*Blurred vision
*Feelings of panic

*Sudden anger
*Crying and weeping
*Leg Cramps
*Running eyes
*Flu and colds
*Bruise easily
*Back aches
*Fibroids
*Lack of appetite
*Infertility
*Boils
*Joint swelling
*Hysteria
*Dry skin
*Insomnia
*Bloating
*Inflammation
*Gall bladder problems
*Slow digestion

Estrogen deficiency or an imbalance of the hormone, can cause:
*Vaginal dryness
*Anxiety
*Mood swings
*Sagging skin
*Poor sleep quality

*Memory problems
*Fatigue
*Lethargy
*Depression
*Night sweats
*Hot flashes
*Painful intercourse
*Bladder infections.
On the other side, estrogen excess can cause:
*Low blood sugar
*Salt and fluid retention
*Foggy thought process
*Migraine tension headaches
*Heavy blood flow
*Puffing and bloating in the body
*Rapid weight gain
*Depression
*Anxiety
*Insomnia
*Hair loss
*Weight gain
*Headaches
*Fatty breasts
*Enlarged prostate
Progesterone deficiency can cause:
*Infertility
*Sleep disorder
*Weight gain
*Miscarriages
*PMS symptoms
*Mood swings
*Anxiety
*Depression
*Painful breasts, lumpy breasts
*Endometriosis
*Breast Cancer

*Tumors
*Osteoporosis
*Water retention
*Depressed libido
Androgen--Male Hormone Dominance can cause:
*Thinning hair
*Unusual facial hair on the face as well as arms and legs
*Acne break outs
*Hypoglycemia
*Tumors
*Osteoporosis
*Water retention
*Depressed libido.
A cortisol imbalance is a stress hormone imbalance causing:
*Fatigue
*Blood sugar issues
*Increased insulin levels
*Weight gain
*Thin dry skin
*Brown age spots, including on the face
*Inability to exercise
When testosterone deficiency is present there is:
*Weight gain
*Fatty breasts
*Soft erections
*Low libido
*Loss of muscle
*Loss of stamina

If you have any of these

above symptoms of hormonal imbalance and you'd like to increase your energy levels, experience a higher quality of sleep, or get your fat burning hormones to work for you instead of against you, the programs we offer at Club Reduce can help you to become balanced and get back to the lifestyle you enjoyed in the past.

Designing the correct hormone program for you will be determined by completing the symptom assessment that we discussed in Chapter Four. After an evaluation we'll be able to determine which supplementation would be beneficial for you. The supplementation would likely include products such as wild yam cream, Hormone Balance and DHEA.

Hormone Balance

Other than starting on a nutritional program and eating the correct and healthy way--which was covered in depth in Chapter Two--we often recommend Hormone Balance by Solutions4. Hormone Balance has been developed to be the most complete hormonal stabilizer ever formulated for both women and men. Hormones are chemicals secreted by the glands in the body. Once a hormone is released into the blood stream it circulates to a target gland. The hormone acts as a messenger instructing the target gland to make its own hormone.
The body makes dozens of hormones that regulate functions throughout the body. Some hormones regulate the fighting off of viral and bacterial infections. Others regulate digestion. Others help manage stress and regulate body tension and blood flow. The ovaries, adrenals, pituitary and hypothalamus regulate levels of estrogen, progesterone and androgens.

As we age and our lifestyle affects our immune system, our hormone producing organs and glands are also affected. There becomes a need to change our lifestyle to promote healthy hormone production. The conventional approach to hormone imbalance involves the idea that the hormone imbalance in the human body is purely chemical. However, there are natural remedies that are safe and effective; not only for menopause but for any time the hormones of a woman or a man are out of balance. Plant extracts make molecules that are precursors of both estrogen and progesterone. These extracts are easily converted into appropriate hormones. Plants contain hormones that regulate cell metabolism and growth. Some plant foods contain substantial amounts of sterols that are precursors to estrogen and progesterone. Solutions4 Hormone Balance produces this hormone balance by adding herbal extracts that act as hormone precursors allowing the body to produce its own hormones naturally. To review the ingredients of Hormone Balance, refer to the Supplement Chapter.

Solutions4 Wild Yam Cream

Symptoms of hormonal imbalance that respond to progesterone include headaches, depression, motor coordination problems, greasy hair, aggression, mood swings, fainting spells, irritability, violence, migraines, blurred vision, self inflicted injuries, epilepsy, feelings of panic, other drug excess, frustration, sudden anger, dark circles under the eyes, hypoglycemic joint pain, crying and weeping jags, stiffness, muscle pain, leg and muscle cramps, eye irritation or puffiness, lethargy, runny eyes, asthma, and flu and colds.

All of these symptoms can be improved by increasing progesterone. Progesterone is a key component in the ultimate formation and balance of estrogen and testosterone. Solutions4 Wild Yam cream also contains the highest levels of DHEA on the market. DHEA is the most dominant hormone in the body, known as the mother hormone. The balancing cream with wild yam is a transdermal skin supplement. It is absorbed quickly and is transported to areas of need. The application would be a quarter teaspoon daily applied to soft skin areas of the body, the chest, inside the arms, thighs or stomach. Rotate areas of application for maximum results. This is a great product for patients needing extra help with hormone balance.

DHEA

DHEA stands for dehydroepiandrosterone. DHEA is a steroid hormone produced in the body by the adrenal glands. It is the single most abundant steroid in the human blood stream. It is the mother or precursor hormone because the body readily converts it on demand into active hormones such as estrogen, testosterone, cortisone and progesterone. DHEA seems to be the only hormone that declines with age in both men and women and its decline triggers age related disease.

Why is DHEA important? According to scientists, the decline of DHEA in the body is the most reliable indicator of aging and susceptibility to disease. Most age researchers agree that to retard aging and prevent disease, the DHEA blood levels must be maintained at levels found in people in their 20s. Controlled scientific studies conducted as long as fifty five years ago definitely exhibited some of the most profound age retarding, healing and disease preventing benefits ever seen in a single compound. Recent studies have demonstrated that of 5000 women monitored, those who developed breast cancer had less than 10% the average DHEA levels for their age group. Those with above average DHEA levels remained cancer free.

In testing, DHEA levels were dramatically lower in males with premature heart disease than in healthy males. Two hundred and forty two men, ages 50-79, followed for twelve years, all experienced declining DHEA levels. Those with the lowest levels showed the highest history of heart disease. Postmenopausal women with rheumatoid arthritis have significantly low DHEA levels. Women with bone density loss have declining levels of DHEA. People suffering from Alzheimer's disease had a 48% less DHEA level in their body than the control group of the same age.

A study at Temple University School of Medicine found that elevated levels of DHEA caused weight loss without a change in appetite. This is not weight loss due to a breakdown of lean muscle or fluid loss. DHEA appears to create a stabilizing effect on all body systems. It has been found to help overweight people to lose fat and underweight people to gain weight. Calories convert to heat rather than get stored as fat. DHEA helps the body to build lean muscle tissue. DHEA may be the most significant natural weight stabilization supplement ever to be introduced in holistic health.

Current research and studies show that DHEA may be beneficial in preventing and treating diabetes, heart disease, obesity, cancer, auto immune disease, AIDS, Fibroidmyalgia, chronic fatigue syndrome, aging, osteoporosis, rheumatoid arthritis, lupus, multiple sclerosis, Parkinson's Disease, PMS, menopausal symptoms and the elimination of many age related disease. Most patients studied in a double blind study noticed enhanced wellbeing and more energy as well as better clarity of thought, also common was an increase in libido.

When DHEA is swallowed it is first absorbed from the stomach and intestines, then goes through the liver before making its way to the rest of the body. DHEA is first metabolized by the liver.

THE THYROID

Thyroid hormones perform a ton of functions in your body. They help control the amount of oxygen each cell uses, the rate at which your body burns calories, your heart rate, overall growth, body temperature, fertility, digestion, memory and mood.

Every cell in the body has receptor sites for thyroid hormones. The thyroid hormones are responsible for the most basic and fundamental aspects of physiology and the basal metabolic rate. The lack of ideal thyroid hormone leads to the global decline in cellular function of all bodily systems. Disorders for thyroid function are very prevalent in the United States population and continue to increase every year.

Thyroid hormones, especially Synthroid, have been on the top ten most prescribed medications for decades. Hypothyroidism is the most common cause of thyroid dysfunction. The thyroid gland is also very vulnerable to imbalances of the endocrine system. Hormones such as estrogen, progesterone, cortisol and testosterone have major influences on thyroid peridoxate enzymes and thyroid binding globulins as well as thyroid receptor site sensitivities. Many times other endocrine imbalances are the culprit in thyroid imbalances and restoring these imbalances has the greatest promise in supporting thyroid metabolism dysfunction.

The thyroid gland is very vulnerable to environmental disruptors. Many of these known environmental disruptors act as goitrogens and compete with iodine uptake. Environmental insults in combination with iodine deficiency affect symptoms as well. Thyroid physiology is very vulnerable to cross reactions with medications. Hypothyroidism is a cause for a change in energy, mood swings, as well as weight gain.

Your pituitary gland creates thyroid stimulating hormone, TSH, to kick start the thyroid. The thyroid then grabs iodine out of your blood, which hopefully has the correct levels of iodine due to the healthy diet you incorporated after reading Chapter Two. The thyroid grabs iodine from your blood and turns into thyroid hormones. T4, thyroxin, is converted to T3, metabolizing boosting thyroid hormone. This is also done through the liver. 70-80% of the conversion process of T4 to T3, is done through the liver. This is if you have a healthy liver. The liver is only as healthy as what you eat, because your liver is constantly processing digestion, and eliminating toxins. So the more healthy your liver is, the better your transition of T4 to T3 will be.

When you're not eating enough calories, the pituitary gland stops producing enough TSH. The thyroid doesn't produce T4. Less T4 leads to less T3; and less T3 means a slower metabolism. Therefore thyroid hormones get imbalanced, either too high or too low. Chemical reactions all over the body get thrown off. An underactive thyroid can lower energy and make you gain weight. This is called hypothyroidism. As you recall from Chapter Four on Candida, Candida is also a toxic side effect from the ethanol and acetaldehyde affects how the thyroid hormone functions. By clearing up the Candida and eliminating yeast from your diet, the thyroid function from T4 to T3 can have astounding recovery and effect.

ADRENAL GLANDS

The adrenal glands are located in the abdominal area. The adrenal glands sit on top of your kidneys. This is where norepinephrine, epinephrine, and cortisol are produced. The adrenal glands cortisol, also called hydrocortisone, is produced in the adrenal cortex, the outer part of each adrenal gland. The inner part of the adrenal gland, the adrenal medulla, produces the other primary stress hormones, norepinephrine, which restricts blood vessels and increases blood pressure; and epinephrine, which increases heart rate and blood flow to muscles.

Each of these stress hormones is released in different ratios based on the challenges you face in your life. If you're looking at a challenge that you think you can handle, your adrenals release norepinephrine. After you succeed, after you handle the challenge, you release more testosterone, which has a positive effect on the body.

If you face a challenge that seems more difficult, something you're not sure you can handle or masters, then you release more epinephrine. This is also called an anxiety hormone. When you're overwhelmed, totally discouraged and you're convinced that you cannot handle this, you release more cortisol.

Epinephrine and cortisol impact metabolism. When you first become stressed, norepinephrine will tell your body to stop producing insulin so that you can have plenty of fast acting blood glucose ready. Epinephrine will relax the muscles of the stomach and intestines and decrease blood flow to these organs. There is a change in what's called sympathetic to the parasympathetic nervous system. Sympathetic is fight or flight. You're ready to go. Parasympathetic is you're just sitting there after a big meal and your digestive tract is working to digest your food.

These two actions cause some of the high blood sugar and stomach problems associated with stress. Once the stressor has passed, cortisol tells the body to stop producing these hormones and to resume digestion. Cortisol continues to have a huge impact on your blood sugar, particularly on how your body uses fuel.

A catabolic hormone--which is a tearing down hormone, not a building up hormone--cortisol tells your body when fat, protein and carbohydrates are present to burn and when to burn them, depending on what kind of challenge you face. Cortisol can either take your fat in the form of triglycerides and move it to your muscles or break down muscle and convert it to glycogen for more energy. If you haven't released the excess cortisol in your blood by exercising cortisol will increase your cravings for high fat, high carb foods. Once you eat, your body releases a cascade of rewarding brain chemicals that can set up an addictive relationship with food. You feel stressed. You eat. You feel better.

If you don't consciously avoid this pattern you can become physically and psychologically dependent on that release to manage stress. It's no coincidence that stress eating is on the rise. When stress continues for a long time and cortisol levels remain high, the body actually resists weight loss. Cortisol turns adipose sites, young fat cells, into mature fat cells. So when you have stress on your body, chronic overstimulation of our adrenals becomes an epidemic. We are victims of, and addicted to, stress and our bodies pay the price. Long term activation of the stress system has a lethal effect on the body. When you abuse your adrenals as much as we do, you set yourself up for heart disease, diabetes, strokes, and other potentially fatal conditions. Adrenal fatigue can also create insomnia, weight gain, depression, hair loss and carb cravings.

The program at Club Reduce will show you how the increased adrenal stress will increase blood sugar levels in the body, which increases insulin response, which is going to increase fat retention. When you fill out the symptom assessment from Club Reduce we will know and determine how significant the adrenal stress is. We have supplementation for the thyroid as well as the adrenal gland; and we'll be able to review that with you on your first visit.

GROWTH HORMONE

Growth hormone, sometimes called HGH, is one of those hormones that we all want more of. It seems to make things better in our bodies. It helps build muscles, burn fat, helps with heart disease, protects your bones, increases overall health and some say even make you happier. People with higher levels of growth hormone also live longer according to studies.

Don't start taking HCG without getting first tested. One of the primary goals of our program is to increase your natural production of growth hormone; which is entirely possible. Growth hormone is produced in the pituitary gland underneath the hypothalamus and it's one of the most influential anabolic hormones. Anabolic hormones are the hormones that produce muscle, playing a huge role in the growth of bone and other body tissue.

Growth hormone increases your muscle mass in several ways-- by absorbing amino acids, synthesizing them into the muscle and prevents the muscle from breaking down. All of this can raise your resting metabolic rate and give you more power for your exercise and workouts. Growth hormone is an amazing thing to tap into if you're overweight, especially if you have extra fat stores. Fat cells have growth hormone receptors that trigger your cells to break down and bring triglycerides. Growth hormone also discourages your fat cells from absorbing and holding onto any fat floating around in your blood stream. Growth hormone actually counters the insulin's ability to shuttle glucose into the cells and this can also be found by taking the test to determine if Candida is present. If Candida is present it can affect glucose and how glucose is introduced into the cells.

Growth hormone can literally be the most amazing thing available to help you with weight loss. Growth hormone is released a few times throughout the day but the most abundant release of growth hormone is during sleep, usually about one to two hours after falling sleep--around midnight to two o'clock in the morning when you are in deep REM sleep, stage four sleep. This is when growth hormone is released in the largest abundance.

Another way we suppress our growth hormone levels is when we eat too many low quality carbs, refined carbs and processed carbs. This keeps our blood sugar and insulin levels high. Protein, on the other hand, can help with growth hormone production. New evidence is also starting to show that hormones from other animal products with pesticides and other contaminants in our environment and diet can affect and impact our growth hormone levels negatively.

One way to increase our growth hormone is with intense exercise. During intense exercise and interval training, our body will use fat as fuel. I have patients who do exercise, but aren't seeing the results they want from it because they are not incorporating interval training. They are not stressing the body out enough to release any of this growth hormone.

Again, when you exercise it keeps your blood glucose level stable so that you have the energy to keep exercising. When you don't exercise and your muscles become insulin resistant, you increase your level of circulating insulin and you suppress growth hormone even further. When you have circulating insulin the body goes into fat storing mode, not fat burning mode

Our office recommends a supplement from Solutions4 for adrenal support and for stress. This supplement is also used and taken after exercise. The shakes that are also available from Solutions4, in chocolate, vanilla, orange cream and strawberry, are also a really good post recovery workout drink due to the fact that it does have the amino acids, the enzymes, the minerals and twenty grams of protein to help repair the muscles and joints that were just stressed. This is a good source for recovery.

As you can see, hormone regulation and balance are very important for optimal body function and weight loss. In most instances hormones can be regulated with a healthy diet, exercise and natural supplementation.

C H A P T E R

S I X

The Stress Solution

The Stress Solution

Stress has been called the most pervasive malady of our time. The constant pressure associated with living in a fast-paced world has created an environment where almost everyone suffers from stress.

Stress comes at you from every aspect of your life. Your home life is a complex balance between fragile family relationships, household duties, career, and finances. In your work life you must deal with unreasonable customers, equipment breakdowns, uncooperative co-workers, stalled traffic, an impossible-to-please boss, and grueling deadlines. At the same time, the media offers up daily doses of violence, terrorism, natural disasters, political and corporate scandals, and a host of horrors beyond imagining.

Sure we can say to ourselves, pull yourself together, or get a grip, but if it were that easy we wouldn't be feeling anxious or stressed in the first place. Once stress gets its hooks in you, it can turn into a vicious cycle of health issues including headaches, insomnia, anxiety, depression, indigestion, irritable bowel syndrome, chronic fatigue syndrome, fibromyalgia, allergies, and weight gain, all of which cause more stress!

So what is stress anyway?

Stress is an intangible; it's not something you can point to and say, "There, over there, that's stress." You can't go to the corner drug store and ask the pharmacist for a quart of stress. So stress isn't real. It's a symptom of cause and effect.

It may surprise you to know that the circumstances of our lives don't determine our level of stress. Our reaction to circumstances is what dictates the amount of stress we experience. Therefore, stress is not something that happens to us; rather, it happens through us. In other words, stress is something we create in our own lives.

When the human body is healthy, it's in a state of homeostasis, which means it's in a continuous stable condition. Stress disrupts homeostasis and is usually triggered by distressing or fear-related experiences, either real or imagined.

How often do you complain about that aching shoulder, pain in your neck, nagging headache, or upset in your stomach? Before you shrug it off as "just stress," think again. Stress typically shows up at your weakest point, though it actually affects your entire body. Long-term stress can make you old before your time or, worse yet, can make you ill. Not a single part of your body is safe from stress's devastating effects—the heart, brain, muscles, immune system, joints—every single cell of your body is affected by stress, making you vulnerable to illness, disease, pain and weight gain.

Some people are born with the ability to remain calm in a stress-filled world. This chapter is for the rest of us—those of us who need help to relax, revitalize, and rejuvenate. It's also for those of us who want to stay positive in a world filled with negativity. In the upcoming pages, we'll discuss in more detail how stress can harm your body and make it next to impossible for you to lose weight. Then we'll go over an exciting new technology that can protect your body and mind from the ravages of stress.

Stress – Silent, but Deadly

When we encounter stress, it causes a physical reaction known as the fight-or-flight response. This response is hard wired into our brains. It signals the body to fight or flee and is part of the genetic wisdom that protects us from physical harm. This fight-or-flight response starts a sequence of nerve cell firings and chemical releases that prepare our body to either run or fight.

The release of chemicals into the bloodstream, like adrenaline, noradrenalin and cortisol creates a dramatic physical change. Respiratory rate increases. Blood is directed away from the digestive tract and into muscles and limbs where added energy is needed to run or fight. The pupils dilate and sight sharpens. Awareness intensifies and impulses quicken. The perception of pain diminishes. In other words, the body prepares itself—physically and mentally—for fight-or-flight.

Throughout early human development the fight-or-flight response was critical to survival. When a caveman encountered a man-eating tiger, he needed the energy and intensified awareness to fight off the animal or run away.

In our modern world filled with high-pressure jobs, traffic, family challenges, and financial concerns, but very few wild tigers, the fight-or-flight response is rarely triggered by actual physical danger. Instead, worry and anxiety prompt most instances of fight-or-flight today.

By its very nature, the fight-or-flight response bypasses the logical left-brain. This is because our early ancestors didn't have time for a logical debate when a man-eating tiger was a few feet away licking its chops. In today's world, however, bypassing the logical mind can cause distorted thinking and exaggerated feelings of anxiety or fear.

Researchers are now finding that when there is a collective buildup of stress hormones that are not properly metabolized over time, toxicity and disorders of the autonomic nervous system can occur, often resulting in chronic illnesses such as migraine headaches, irritable bowel syndrome, or high blood pressure. Chronic stress also puts you at higher risk for disorders of the hormonal and immune systems, resulting in weight gain, chronic fatigue, depression, and diseases such as rheumatoid arthritis, lupus, allergies and, yes, even cancer.

You may be thinking, "I really never feel that stressed out." This is because excess stress doesn't always show up as the feeling of being stressed. Stress often goes directly to the body and may only be recognized by the symptoms it creates such as weight gain, headaches, depression, anxiety, or disease.

You might even be using food as medicine to deal with this excess stress. We'll discuss this further later in the chapter.

How Does Stress Affect Your Body?

As I mentioned earlier, stress is not something that happens to us, it is something we create in our own lives based on how we react to circumstances. Let's take a look at some of the physical responses your body can have to stress, how getting overwhelmed affects your health, and why reducing stress is so essential to your well-being.

Stress Effect #1: The Heart

Whenever the fight-or-flight response is triggered, whether through real or imagined stress, an increase in heart rate, blood pressure, and breathing delivers more oxygen faster throughout the body. At the same time, a rapid release of glucose and fatty acids into the bloodstream occurs. This is how your body can respond with strength and stamina during an emergency.

Chronic stress, however, can lead to high blood pressure and undue strain on the heart. The added glucose, if unused by the body, can cause elevated or erratic blood sugar levels. These blood sugar swings can make you feel fatigued and can lead to diabetes. Stress also prompts the body to release cortisol, which can cause a build up of cholesterol in the arteries. The bottom line: Stress can contribute to cardiovascular disease.

Stress Effect #2: The Brain

Are you one of those people who work best on deadlines? Do you use stress as a motivator? If so, you may be doing long-term harm to your brain that could cause early memory loss or may even lead to Alzheimer's.

You may thrive on stress because of the short-term brain boost of glucose your brain gets when you're under the gun. When this happens, your senses are heightened and your memory improves. Problems start when stress lasts more than two hours. That's when the body assumes you need more physical strength than brainpower and starts sending the glucose back to the muscles, leaving your brain short of glucose. At the same time, stress hormones impair neuron functioning. Another part of the brain, the hippocampus, associated with learning and memory, can get smaller over time due to the loss of glucose and damage to neurons. Researchers don't know the full effect of a shrinking hippocampus, but they do know that it can make you forgetful and muddle your thinking.

Stress Effect #3: The Immune System

Whenever the fight-or-flight response is triggered, stress hormones course through your body and signal the non-essential functions to stop or slow down so that all systems essential to dealing with an emergency receive an extra boost of energy. Your immune system is not required for urgent activity. Therefore, it temporarily stops or slows down during peak stress periods. This system works out fine when the stress is short term, but when the stress hormones keep pouring in, your immune system suffers, making you vulnerable to infection, inflammation (which translates to weight gain) and disease.

Stress Effect #4: Body Fat

I once wrote an article called, "Why Stress is More Fattening than Chocolate." During my years of running weight loss clinics, I heard client after client ask me, "Why is it that my friends can gobble up everything in sight and not gain a pound, while I nibble on salads and the scale won't budge?"

With a little research, I found the answer in a powerful hormone called cortisol. Cortisol's job is to signal the body to relax and refuel after periods of stress; it's the body's way of slowing us down so that we don't burn out. After reviewing my client files, I realized that almost everyone who complained that he or she couldn't lose weight, even while dieting, lived with at least one high-stress factor that was likely causing high cortisol levels.

Cortisol's message to slow down tends to make us feel tired, lethargic, and hungry. Therefore, while under the powerful influence of cortisol, our tendency is to want to lie around, watch television, and snack, thus the term, stress-eater, and the reason stress can be more fattening than chocolate.

Cortisol also triggers fat storage in the adipose tissue of the abdomen. When the majority of weight is in the abdomen it gives one an apple appearance. More importantly, it can lead to Cushing's Syndrome, which involves storage of fat on the inside of the abdominal cavity. Cushing's Syndrome can be dangerous and may lead to diabetes and heart disease.

What is the Relationship Between Hormones and Stress?

Anti-aging specialists now know that hormone levels are affected by two factors: aging and stress. While we can't do much about the ticking clock, we certainly can control our stress factors. When hormone levels drop, the diseases regularly associated with aging appear. These diseases, including obesity, heart attack, stroke, osteoporosis, cancer, and dementia are all accepted as the natural ravages of aging. Studies on aging, however, now show that we can greatly reduce our risk of these diseases by reducing the level of stress in our lives.

Have you ever noticed how some people seem to get old before their time, or were you ever shocked to hear about a thirty-eight year old having a fatal heart attack? In all likelihood, their bodies were the victims of chronic stress that depleted their hormones and forced their bodies into early aging.

Most people are familiar with the sex hormones, estrogen, progesterone, and testosterone, but few are aware of the hormones that drive the metabolism and affect body weight.

Thyroid Hormones

Blood circulation, body temperature, metabolism, and brain function are all driven by thyroid hormones. Energy levels and sex drive are influenced by thyroid hormones as well. When the thyroid is working optimally, it protects against heart disease and strokes, lowers cholesterol, improves brain metabolism, and helps prevent memory problems. When the body is too frequently in fight-or-flight mode, the thyroid function can decrease, or in some instances may stop producing hormones.

Insulin

Almost everyone knows someone who developed Type II diabetes later in life. Type II diabetes is called a lifestyle disease because it is caused by lifestyle choices, such as poor diet, lack of exercise, obesity, and chronic stress. Appropriate lifestyle changes can prevent or even reverse Type II diabetes.

When the hormone insulin is depleted, the result is Insulin Resistance Syndrome (IRS). Gone unchecked, IRS can quickly turn into diabetes, or it may lead to other serious health conditions such as high blood pressure, abnormal cholesterol or triglycerides, stroke, and gout.

Cortisol

Cortisol has recently been touted as the new wonder weight loss remedy. Because low cortisol levels can lead to fat storage, the assumption is that if you stimulate the body to produce more cortisol, you'll lose weight. This is a dangerous assumption.

Most people don't realize that cortisol is a hormone produced naturally by the body, or that stress is what caused its depletion in the first place. Cortisol is the body's stress management system, but it has its limits.

Cortisol is secreted by the adrenals, tiny glands located just above each kidney. Don't let the adrenal glands' diminutive size fool you. The hormones produced here are absolutely essential to human life. For instance, when my sister-in-law's lung cancer spread to her adrenal glands, she struggled even to lift her fingers.

Powerful steroids extended her life by a few months, but the reality is, too many of her body's systems required the important hormones secreted by the adrenal glands. Our bodies simply can't function without these hormones, especially cortisol.

Chronic or acute states of fight-or-flight increase the body's cortisol secretion. When cortisol levels are high, it can actually lead to weight gain because cortisol is your body's signal to slow down. Other symptoms may include anxiety, mental fogginess, insomnia, and high blood pressure. If this goes on for too long, the body's stores of cortisol become depleted and adrenal fatigue sets in—a weak immune system, depression, weight gain and chronic fatigue result.

DHEA

DHEA is another stress-reactive hormone secreted by the adrenal glands. When secreted at proper levels, it aids in lowering cholesterol, thus reducing the risk of heart attacks and stroke. DHEA also helps to reduce body fat, stimulates the metabolism and immune systems, maintains sexual vitality, and boosts the mood. Considered an anti-stress hormone, DHEA can help prevent anxiety and depression.

Melatonin

Melatonin, the hormone associated with sleep patterns, influences the body's ability to rejuvenate and repair. It is secreted by the pineal gland, located at the base of the brain. Melatonin is produced from serotonin, the hormone associated with mood. You'll learn more about serotonin in the next section. When high stress levels disturb sleep, the production of melatonin is inhibited, the immune system is compromised, and the rejuvenation and repair of cells is impaired. During the deeper sleep stages, the body produces natural killer cells—the cells that devour cancers and other free radicals in the body. Insufficient or depleted melatonin can put you at higher risk of developing cancer or other immune deficiency diseases. Additionally, melatonin deficits can result in irritability and premature aging.

As you can see, chronic stress can cause early depletion of nearly every hormone your body produces. And depletion of hormones equates to weight gain or the inability to shed weight, early aging and disease.

The good news is that you can learn to quiet your mind, calm your body, and directly overcome the harmful effects of the fight-or-flight response—you will, in fact, gain the healthy benefits of its opposite—the relaxation response.

Lose Your Stress, Lose Your Weight

The doctors at Club Reduce are always on the lookout for health breakthroughs and new technology that can help patients not only take off pounds and inches quickly and easily, but also realize optimum health. When Dr. Singleton called me about using Self-Mastery Technology (SMT) with his already proven Club Reduce program, we knew we were onto something big.

Even as Dr. Singleton's Club Reduce program was getting amazing results for patients, he recognized that there was still one missing link to the optimum health equation—the mind. He had witnessed hundreds of patients who were smart and confident in every other aspect of their lives, who displayed tremendous self-control in their careers and home life, yet when it came to food, were completely out of control.

Why were these intelligent, capable people so controlled by food?

Research conducted by Dr. David Kessler, the scientist who once led the U.S. government's attack on addictive cigarettes, may have found one clue. Dr. Kessler recently published research suggesting that millions of Americans increasingly share a new malady he calls conditioned hyper-eating, a willpower-sapping drive to eat—especially high-fat, high-sugar foods—even when not hungry.

This condition occurs in the brain where these foods light up the brain's dopamine (pleasure-sensing) pathway—the same pathway that conditions people to alcohol or drugs. According to Kessler, this factor is one of the root causes of the obesity epidemic in our country today.

If at times you feel as if you're a slave to food, you may already be a victim to this devastating condition. Symptoms include:

- Feeling that food controls you
- Eating even when you're not hungry
- Eating too fast
- Craving sugar, salt and fat
- Eating without conscious awareness (such as finishing a whole bag of chips without remembering to taste or enjoy them)
- Feeling compelled to continue eating even when you know you should stop
- The inability to identify the feeling of fullness
- The ability to relieve anxiety or depression by eating

If you experience any of these symptoms, your brain has likely already developed conditioned hyper-eating. It's a form of self-medicating (or relieving stress) with food and it's fast becoming the leading health threat in the U.S. and around the globe. Kessler says overeaters must, "retrain their brains to resist the lure." He suggests that overcoming conditioned hyper-eating takes vigilant discipline and self-control.

But didn't he just say lack of self-control is the problem? How can the problem also be the solution?

Fortunately, there is an easier way. You can retrain your brain to eliminate conditioned hyper-eating, end stress-eating, and put a halt to emotional eating—minus the grueling discipline.

It's a proven form of brainwave training that I've been using for decades with exciting results for thousands of clients. The system uses gentle pulses of light and sound in combination with guided Self-Mastery Technology (SMT) audio-sessions. This form of brainwave entrainment, combined with mind messaging (also known as creative visualization), works by retraining your dopamine pathways while "re-programming" your thoughts and emotions relating to food, health, and self-esteem.

After all, what good would it do for you to lose all your weight only to fall back into the habit of conditioned hyper-eating that caused your weight problem in the first place?

So you see, to achieve weight loss for life, you not only must take off your excessive weight, but also have the right mind-set, correct eating habits and the positive, stress-free lifestyle necessary for keeping your weight off for a lifetime.

While you read through Weight Loss For Life you are learning about your body and how to optimize it with nutrition, but now you know there is also a need to retrain your mind.

High-Tech Solutions for Stress

Self-Mastery Technology using light and sound frequencies is also known as visual/auditory entrainment. The user wears head-phones and special glasses equipped with LED lights. The lights flash at predetermined frequencies and are coupled with binaural beats, which are heard at a low level through the headphones. The visual/auditory entrainment is typically synchronized, but can be varied depending on the desired effect.

The flickering light patterns and binaural beats reach the brain by way of the optic nerve and inner ear respectively. Within minutes the brain begins to match the frequencies of the light pulses and sound beats. The method by which this entrainment occurs is known as frequency following response. Unlike biofeedback, where the user attempts to consciously change brainwave activity, light and sound induced entrainment influences the brain without any conscious effort.

The frequency following response simulates the relaxed brainwave frequencies know as alpha and theta.

This is the state in which the individual relaxes and the mind develops focus. Listeners experience a reduction in inner chatter and improved concentration. Because frequency following response is a learned response, the effect is cumulative. After a few weeks of regular use, users gain a sense of balance and inner calm. Most people report feeling serene, focused, and alert even when faced with high-pressure situations. Furthermore, most users report experiencing enhanced creativity and they feel more rested with less sleep.

Self-Mastery Technology or SMT uses four very distinct processes and each one on their own is very powerful. When combined, these technologies form a powerful matrix to help super-charge the body-mind connection so that you can easily access the resources you need to create lasting change in your life.

Self-Mastery Technology #1
Brainwave Entrainment Tones

How Binaural Beats Work

1. The binaural beat is generated from two separate tones of a slightly different pitch

2. One tone is presented to the left ear and the other to the right ear

3. Your brain combines the two tones to make a single new tone

4. The single tone pulses to match relaxed brainwave frequencies

5. Your brain follows the pattern and creates the relaxed state

In 1839, an associate professor at the University of Berlin discovered what he termed binaural beats. His early research showed that putting a given frequency in one ear and a different tone in the other causes a person to hear a third tone, which is the difference in frequency of the two tones.

He found that the human ability to hear binaural beats appeared to be the result of evolutionary adaptation and that our brains detect and follow binaural beats because of the structure of the brain itself.

Self-Mastery Technology #2
Frequency Following Response (FFR)

Four Brainwave Frequencies

Brainwave Frequency	Name

13–40 Hz   *Beta waves (Reactionary Mind)*
Active thought and concentration; associated with busyness and anxious thinking

7–13 Hz   *Alpha waves (Intuitive Mind)*
Relaxation (while awake), daydreaming; associated with creativity

4–7 Hz   *Theta waves (Inventive Mind)*
The place between asleep and awake; associated with deep meditation and sleep learning

< 4 Hz   *Delta waves (Rejuvenating Mind)*
Deep dreamless sleep

Almost since the time humans discovered fire, it's been observed that flickering light can cause alterations in consciousness. Early scientists, captivated by this phenomenon, explored its practical applications.

By 1990, scientists were able to measure the effect of light on serotonin and endorphin levels. In one such study, eleven patients had peridural (the outermost of the three membranes covering the brain and spinal cord) and blood analysis performed before and after participation in relaxation sessions using flash emitting goggles. An average increase of beta-endorphin levels of twenty-five percent and serotonin levels of twenty-one percent were registered. The beta-endorphin levels are comparable to those obtained by cranial electrical stimulation (CES). The researchers concluded that photic stimulation has great potential for decreasing depression-related symptoms.

Self-Mastery Technology #3

Alpha Learning Music

Ever since the dawn of civilization, man has recognized the profound effect of music on human behavior and learning. The ancient Greeks believed that music was divinely created. Both Plato and Aristotle placed music at the core of their educational curricula, acknowledging music's power to stimulate human thought and understanding.

Club Reduce tapped into modern research, which has given us scientific explanations for the 'magic' of music that the ancients recognized by instinct and observation. Today, there is no doubt that music has a powerful impact on almost every aspect of the body and mind of the listener.

As a therapist, teacher and a parent, I have been interested in discovering methods by which my students might use music as an aid to learning faster and more efficiently. For more than four decades my father, Dr. Michael Porter, and I have been recommending background music as a key element in the application of super-learning. It started with the study of the "Silva Method" and Jose Silva's "Alpha Sound."

Research around the relationship between super-learning and music focused on the Baroque style. However, modern artist like Alexander and Steven Halpern have used a mix of computer generated music and classic melodies to create a powerful mix of alpha music that is used in the Club Reduce Self-Mastery Technology sessions.

Self-Mastery Technology #4
Creative Visualizations

What is Mind Messaging?

Mind messaging is a form of guided visualization used to help the listener form positive mental images. Visualization it is the primary component of the imagination and is at the core of the human ability to create, innovate and dream.

Many of history's inventors and artists attribute their success to an exceptional ability to visualize. Thomas Edison, Nikola Tesla, Henry Ford and the great composer, Chopin all reported using creative visualization to spark their imaginations. Additionally, Albert Einstein once said that he came up with the theory of relativity by imagining what would happen if he could travel through space on the tip of a light beam.

Mind messaging utilizes the language of the mind to transport you out of a state of stress or fear, and into a new space of inner calm, peace and tranquility where you can easily change habits and behaviors. Additionally, a natural byproduct of this form of visualization occurs when the body goes loose and limp, thereby creating the relaxation response—the perfect state for learning, healing, or focusing on goals.

We all have an inner critic, a part of our mind that, based on past experience, will reject unfamiliar information without proper evaluation. This is known as the critical factor. Studies have shown that relaxation techniques subdue this critical factor, and make you receptive to new ideas. Even though it may seem counterintuitive to "let go in order to gain control," this is exactly what happens during the relaxation response.

Through mind messaging techniques, you experience positive and appropriate ways to imagine your personal goals. This helps you remain optimistic and motivated toward the changes that bring about your success.

Mind/Body Healing

Visualization has long been the primary tool for mind/body healing. From a scientific perspective, we know that, because visualization directly impacts the body's neurological system, it can have a direct influence on us physically.

Try this for an example. Imagine I have just handed you a large, yellow, juice-filled lemon. You slice the lemon into quarters and bring one of the quarters to your mouth and bite into it...what happened? Did your mouth begin to pucker? Did it fill with saliva? This is a naturally occurring neurological response to an imagined thought.

Have you ever watched a horror film and, in the midst of the excitement, found that your palms were sweating and your heart was pounding? You knew it was "just a movie," though, right?

If your mind can cause this kind of impact on the body, is there any reason it can't relax your muscles, overpower nicotine, stimulate your metabolism, release unwanted fat, do away with chronic pain, or even trigger the immune system to eliminate cancer cells?

Together, we can change your mind

I believe the best way, and sometimes the only way, to make changes in your life is to first change your mind. Because images, beliefs, and values are so deeply rooted in consciousness, changes must happen at the other-than-conscious level before they can manifest in your life. In my experience, the combined light/sound/mind messaging used in Self-Mastery Technology is the quickest and easiest way to change your mind.

If you plant a seed, and know that you are watering and caring for it, you can pretty much sit back, relax, and let it sprout. You wouldn't keep digging up the dirt to see if the seed sprouted, would you? If you did uncover the seed to see if it is sprouting, you would probably stop its growth. I believe that this is what happens when people try to make changes at the conscious level; they set a goal, but then find themselves digging up old images, beliefs, and thought patterns, and end up stopping their growth.

When you relax with Self-Mastery Technology guiding your conscious mind, you are free to liberate your other-than-conscious mind. Psychologists would say that you are bypassing the critical factor and letting the other-than-conscious mind take over. In other words, you plant the seeds of change, then sit back, relax, and let them sprout.

What are the Benefits of Self-Mastery Technology?

Whenever people ask me why I'm so passionate about light and sound technology, I tell them one of my favorite jokes. It goes something like this: One evening a man in a tuxedo rushed up to a street musician and asked, "How do you get to Carnegie Hall?" Without skipping a beat the musician answered, "Practice, man, practice!"

SMT works because it involves mental practice or spaced repetition. In my opinion, there is no faster or easier method for achieving spaced repetition than through the synchronized rhythm of light and sound. The induction into higher brainwave states increases brain activity, while the induction of lower brainwave states reduces hyperactivity and feelings of anxiety. In other words, it puts you in the perfect mind state of changing your eating habits and lifestyle.

Research showing the efficacy of light and sound technology is not uncommon. Creative visualization and stimulation of brain wave activity are among the most studied areas of psychiatry and psychology. The following results have been demonstrated through numerous studies and in my own experience with thousands of clients:

- Increased long and short-term memory
- Increased attention span and concentration
- Reduction of anxiety and depression
- Reduction of medication intake
- Increase in right-left visual-spatial integration
- Major increase in creativity idea generation
- Easier decision making and holistic problem solving
- Decrease in migraine or headache frequency and intensity
- Reduction in PMS and menopause symptoms
- Reduction in insomnia and sleep disorders
- Improvement of motivation

All of this is in addition to the benefits of deep relaxation that I outlined earlier. People who regularly use SMT often say, "Things just don't bother me anymore." When it comes to weight loss, this translates to a more positive attitude, enhanced self-control, confidence, and better decision-making.

The Self-Mastery Technology system used at Club Reduce is called the ZenFrames Portable Achievement Device, a proven form of brainwave technology that uses gentle pulses of light and sound delivered through a hand-held device that's smaller than a deck of cards. The device works in combination with mind messaging to "re-pattern" your thoughts, attitudes, and emotions relating to food. People who want to lose weight long-term can relax with this system for just twenty-minutes a day. Listeners regularly report that their eating habits, health, and self-esteem all improve.

It doesn't make any sense to start a diet unless you also have the right mind-set, correct eating habits and the positive, stress-free lifestyle necessary for keeping weight off for a lifetime. Self-Mastery Technology can help you do all that and more.

CHAPTER SEVEN

Blood Sugar Disorders

Chapter 7
Blood Sugar Disorders

In this chapter, we'll talk about diabetes, hypoglycemia, Syndrome X, insulin resistance and unexplained weight gain.

What Is Diabetes?

Diabetes is defined as too much sugar in the blood. Diabetes is a chronic disorder of blood sugar and metabolism--how you body uses food. Having diabetes means you are not able to utilize and break down the food like other people. Normal blood sugar keeps you healthy. Blood sugar should be between 70 and 110.

Too low, below 70, and you will feel shaky and sweaty. Too high, over 150, can make you feel tired and sleepy. Diabetes Mellitus is an ailment that occurs when the pancreas is unable to secrete enough insulin to keep up and maintain a normal blood sugar glucose level, leading to high blood sugar levels.

A person is regarded as having diabetes mellitus if their blood sugar concentration is greater than 140 milligrams per deciliter after an overnight fast. Diabetes can lead to serious complications like kidney failure, heart disease neuropathy and premature death. People with diabetes can take steps to control the disease and lower the risk of complications.

The symptom assessment available at our office, the questionnaire we ask you to fill out when you come in, will help determine if there is a pre-diabetic prevalence in you.

Symptoms of Diabetes

Some of the symptoms of diabetes include frequent urination. This occurs because the body is trying to get rid of the extra blood glucose and this is one way it can be done, through your urine. Because of the frequent urination the body needs to replace the lost water, so you feel thirsty more often. Your body is not able to properly use the foods you do eat, so the body thinks it's not getting enough fuel. Therefore you may feel hungry more often and eat the foods that come out of a box, bag or can to give you quick energy. Also, since the cells in your body are not able to use the sugar properly you may not have energy to carry out your normal activities.

Symptoms of Type I Diabetes may include:

- Frequent urination
- Unusual thirst
- Extreme hunger
- Unusual weight loss
- Extreme fatigue and Irritability

Symptoms of Type II Diabetes may include:

- Any of the type 1 symptoms
- Frequent infections
- Blurred vision
- Cuts/bruises that are slow to heal
- Tingling/numbness in the hands/feet
- Recurring skin, gum, or bladder infections

Be aware, however, that many people with Type II diabetes may show no symptoms at all until the disease is upon you. You may have normal blood values for years until it becomes out of control.

Hypoglycemia (Low Blood Sugar)

Hypoglycemia is a catch-22 disease where insulin counteracts high blood sugar levels leading to low blood sugar, blood glucose, leading to a craving for more sugar. Hypoglycemia is a modern affliction that was not discovered until 1924. It has now become one of the fastest spreading and most prevalent ailments in America today.

Hypoglycemia has no geographical boundaries. It's found in every city and county throughout the United States. It has no age, income or occupational boundaries. It is currently estimated that hypoglycemia affects upwards of 50 million Americans in all walks of life, most of who don't even know they have it. Thousands more are developing it on a daily basis.

I've found in my clinic that by testing patients with the symptom assessment if candida shows up there is a high likelihood of hypoglycemia; and that by restoring the body's communication systems between the cells, the insulin and the blood sugar being able to get to the cells, the blood sugar balances and normalizes. Patients that were Type II diabetics are now using less medication or none at all; and Type

I diabetics have even been shown to use less of their insulin.

Symptoms of hypoglycemia include feeling shaky and weak. The body may be shaky and weak since there is not enough energy for your muscles. Sweating is a common physical response to low blood sugar. Your body is telling you something is wrong. The body will sense the low blood sugar and will signal the brain to try and find something to eat causing feelings of hunger.

You may feel tired because the muscles don't have enough glucose to produce energy leaving you to not function as you normally would. You may be irritable and confused because as the brain uses only glucose for energy. If you don't have enough glucose the brain can't function properly causing irritability and confusion. These symptoms can range depending on the severity of the hypoglycemia involved as seen below:

Mild hypoglycemia

Symptoms of mild low blood sugar usually occur when blood sugar falls below 70 mg/dL and may include:

- Nausea
- Extreme hunger
- Feeling nervous or jittery
- Cold, clammy, wet skin and/ or excessive sweating not caused by exercise
- Rapid heartbeat
- Numbness or tingling of the fingertips or lips
- Trembling

Moderate hypoglycemia

If blood sugar continues to fall, the nervous system can be affected. Symptoms usually occur when the blood sugar falls below 55 mg/dL and may include:

- Mood changes, such as irritability, anxiety, restlessness, or anger
- Confusion, difficulty in thinking, or inability to concentrate
- Blurred vision, dizziness or headache
- Weakness, lack of energy

- Poor coordination
- Difficulty walking or talking, such as staggering or slurred speech
- Fatigue, lethargy, or drowsiness

Severe hypoglycemia

The symptoms of severe low blood sugar develop when blood sugar falls below 35 mg/dL to 40 mg/dL and may include:

- Seizures or convulsions
- Loss of consciousness, coma
- Low body temperature (hypothermia)

Insulin Resistance (Syndrome X)

Syndrome X or insulin resistance is a condition that involves a decrease in the sensitivity of the body's cells to the actions of insulin or a decrease in insulin sensitivity. Insulin resistance is characterized by a decreased sensitivity of insulin receptors for insulin. This lack of sensitivity results in ever increasing production of insulin to the extent that dangerously high levels of insulin can occur.

There is no single laboratory test for the diagnosis of insulin resistance. The diagnosis is based on clinical findings corroborated with laboratory tests. The following testes are often used in conjunction with the clinical findings.

Fasting total cholesterol: high levels may indicate insulin resistance.

Total serum triglycerides: high levels may indicate insulin resistance.

High density lipoproteins: low levels of HDL-C may indicate insulin resistance.

Low density lipoproteins: high levels of LDL-B may indicate insulin resistance.

Uric acid: high uric acid levels may indicate insulin resistance.

Fibrinogen: high.

Homocysteine: High and is an amino acid in the blood. Epidemiological studies have shown that too much homocysteine in the blood (plasma) is related to a higher risk of coronary heart disease, stroke and peripheral vascular disease.

Other evidence suggests that homocysteine may have an effect on atherosclerosis by damaging the inner lining of arteries and promoting blood clots. High levels may also indicate insulin resistance.

Statistics about Diabetes in the United States

The total prevalence of Diabetes in the United States covering all ages as of 2005 totaled 23.6 million people, which is 7% of the population; 17.9 million people included in that number have been diagnosed with this condition; and 5.7 million people have this condition but have not been diagnosed. 25% of the population of the United States has insulin resistance. Every 21 seconds another American is diagnosed with diabetes. About 176,500 of the people diagnosed with diabetes are aged twenty years or younger. This represents .22% the entire population in this age group or about one in every 400-600 children and adolescents with Type I diabetes.

Although Type II diabetes can occur in youth, the nationally representative data that would be needed to monitor the diabetes trends in the youth by type are not available. Clinically based reports and regional studies suggest that Type II diabetes due to diet, is being diagnosed more frequently in children and adolescents, particularly in the ethnic groups including American Indians, African Americans and Hispanic or Latino Americans and anybody else that does not care what they put in their mouth.

Incidence of diabetes in the United States

The incidence of diabetes in this country is on the rise. 1.5 million new cases of diabetes were diagnosed in people aged twenty years or older in 2005. Deaths among people with diabetes in the United States, in 2002 Diabetes was the sixth leading cause of deaths listed on death certificates in 2002. This ranking is based on the 73,249 death certificates in which diabetes was listed as the underlying cause of death. Diabetes contributed to a total of 224,092 deaths. Diabetes is likely to be underreported as a cause of death.

Studies have found that only about 35-40% of decedents with diabetes had it listed anywhere on the death certificate and only about 10-15% had it listed as the underlying cause of death. Overall, the risk for death among people with diabetes is about twice that of people without diabetes of similar age.

Complications of Diabetes in the United States

Heart disease and stroke: Heart disease and stroke account for about 65% of deaths in people who have diabetes. Adults with diabetes have heart disease death rates about two to four times higher than adults without diabetes. The risk for stroke is two to four times higher among people with diabetes.

High Blood Pressure: About 73% of adults with diabetes have blood pressure greater than or equal to 130/80 millimeters of mercury or use prescription medication for hypertension.

Blindness: Diabetes is the leading cause of new cases of blindness among adults aged twenty to seventy years. Diabetic retinopathy causes 12,000-24,000 new cases of blindness each year.

Kidney disease: Diabetes is the leading cause of kidney failure, accounting for 44% of new cases in 2002. In 2002 44,000 people with diabetes began treatment for end stage kidney disease in the United States and Puerto Rico. A total of 153,730 people with end stage kidney disease due to diabetes were living on chronic dialysis or with a kidney transplant in the United States and Puerto Rico.

Nervous System Disease: About 60-70% of people with diabetes have mild to severe forms of nervous system damage. The results of such damage include impaired sensation or pain in the feet or hands, slow digestion of food in the stomach, carpal tunnel syndrome and other nerve problems. Almost 30% of people with diabetes ages 40 and older have impaired sensation in the feet, at least one area that lacks feeling. Severe forms of diabetic nerve disease are a major contributing cause of lower extremity amputations.

I have had patients before who have come in with numbness and tingling in their feet. None of the blood tests they've received have shown any blood sugar issues. Once they've filled out the Club Reduce symptom assessment can I then determined they maybe pre-diabetic.

We can help the symptoms of Diabetes with nutrition and cold laser treatments on the lower extremities that are numb and tingling.

We need to stay on top of this pre-condition with our natural treatment until the body can heal itself.

I had a patient recently, we will call her Brenda, who came in complaining that she had numbness and tingling and hadn't been able to wear shoes. Her doctor had told her if she kept going down this road she'd lose her legs. We discovered she had candida and put her on our twelve week candida program. She lost fifty five pounds in three and now can wear shoes. She has gone from a size 4X to an XL. She has no more neuropathy and no more numbness and tingling due to a changing lifestyle and laser treatments.

Amputation: More than 60% of non traumatic lower limb amputations occur in people with diabetes. In 2002 about 82,000 non traumatic lower limb amputations were performed in people with diabetes.

Dental Disease: Periodontal gum disease is more common in people with diabetes. Among young adults, those with diabetes have about twice the risk of those without diabetes. Almost one third of people with diabetes have severe periodontal disease with loss of attachment of the gums to the teeth measuring five millimeters or more.

Complications in pregnancy: Poorly controlled diabetes before conception and during the first trimester of pregnancy can cause major birth defects in 5 to 10% of pregnancies and spontaneous abortions in 15 to 20% of pregnancies. Poorly controlled diabetes during the second and third trimesters of pregnancy can result in excessively large babies, posing a risk to both mother and child.

Other Complications: Uncontrolled diabetes often leads to biochemical imbalances that can cause acute life threatening events such as diabetic ketoacidosis. People with diabetes are more susceptible to many other illnesses and once they acquire the disease and will have a poor prognosis. For example, they are more likely to die with pneumonia or influenza than people who do not have diabetes.

The Glycemic Index

The glycemic index ranks foods on how they affect our blood glucose levels. A low GI food will cause a small rise, low glycemic. A high GI food will trigger a dramatic spike, high glycemic. A GI that is 70 (On the scale of 1 to 100) or more is high. A GI of 56 to 69 inclusive is medium. A GI of 55 or less is low. A GI under 20 is ultra low. You can slow the rate at which your blood sugar spikes by using the following: Protein, fat, fiber.

When choosing foods it is important to note what nutrients you're getting, what vitamins, minerals, phytochemicals, proteins, carbs, fiber, essential fatty acids. Don't just eat empty calories. When regulating the blood sugar levels through the glycemic index it's best to eat more vegetables and some lean protein to keep the blood sugar levels low and the glycemic index low.

Net Carbohydrates

When looking at how many carbohydrates are in food it's important to look at the net carbs. Net carbs are the total carbohydrates minus the fiber. Fiber does not require insulin for utilization so it is not counted toward carbohydrates that impact your blood sugar.

Glycemic Load - The Bottom Line for Your Blood Sugar

The glycemic load estimates blood sugar response based on how many carbs are in a serving of a food multiplied by its glycemic index. Therefore, the glycemic load, GL, takes the glycemic index into account but provides a more detailed response to the rise in blood sugar. A GL, glycemic index, value specifies how rapidly a particular carbohydrate turns into sugar. It doesn't tell you how much of that carbohydrate is in a serving of a particular food. It is important to know the glycemic load to understand a food's effect on blood sugar. The glycemic load of a food gives you the most accurate number when planning your meals for sustained blood sugar balance.

General Guidelines for the Glycemic Index of Foods
The glycemic index ranges from 0 to 100.

A high glycemic index food would have a score ranging from 71 to 100. Some examples of foods in this category would include simple carbohydrates such as honey, glucose syrup, Maltodextrin, fruit juices, regular sodas, carrot juice and Gatorade; artificial sweeteners such as Splenda and Equal; vegetables such as carrots, parsnips, baked potatoes and instant potatoes; starches such as white bread and white rice.

The medium glycemic index foods have a score ranging from 56 to 70. These foods should be eaten in moderation and balanced with protein, fiber and good fats. Some of these foods include fruits such as oranges, grapes, bananas and raisins; starches such as brown rice, whole wheat, Ezekiel bread, whole grain or whole grain rye, whole wheat, brown rice spaghetti; vegetables such as sweet potatoes, green peas, corn and beets.

The lower glycemic index foods range from 21 to 55. Your diet should consist mostly of low and ultra low glycemic index foods. These foods include fruits such as apples, peaches, cherries, plums, grapefruit and pears; legumes like lentils, kidney beans, and lima beans.

The ultra low glycemic index foods score from 0 to 20 on the glycemic index scale. You should, again, pattern your diet to include mostly foods from the low and ultra low list of glycemic index foods. Some examples of ultra low glycemic foods include nuts such as almonds, peanuts, cashews, pecans and roasted soybeans; berries including strawberries, blueberries, blackberries and raspberries; fruits such as tomatoes.

Protein sources such as turkey, chicken, fish and tofu have no glycemic index. Meat alternatives also have little or no glycemic index. Again, meats should be hormone free and organic whenever possible. Most vegetables have little or no glycemic index so they are very good choices to include in your diet and should be eaten more than fruit. Your diet should contain 70-80% vegetables compared to 10-20% fruit.

The Solutions4 instant meal is a great source of low glycemic loads on the body and tastes great.

Exercise

There are many good ways to exercise or be active for longer periods of time. Walking is one of the best, as is swimming, dancing, riding bikes or doing other hard work as forms of exercise activity. The best type of exercise activity for you is one that you will do consistently. You can do different types of exercise on different days to keep your motivation alive.

To judge if you're exercising at the correct intensity check how hard you're breathing. You should not be breathing hard enough that you can't talk while exercising.

Exercise is most beneficial if you can get at least a half an hour or more every day of the week. Be aware it may take a while to work up to that point. Start with five minutes a day and slowly increase your activity level as the week's progress.

At Club Reduce we have a diabetic program for those of you who have Type I or Type II diabetes. We also will rule out candida before we begin you on any other program. If you have candida we will recommend the candida program first, which usually balances the blood sugar levels in your body. This can all be determined when you fill out the questionnaire at our office.

CHAPTER
EIGHT

9 Things You must Do TO
Keep Your Body in Fat Burning

CHAPTER EIGHT
9 Steps to Trigger the Fat Burning Hormones in your Body
-- And what to Avoid

THINGS TO AVOID

1. *Starvation.* To maximize fat burning you should avoid allowing your body to reach starvation mode. This happens when you find yourself not eating throughout the day. People are nutritionally starving themselves because they're in a hurry, have no time or are not hungry. Not eating enough can also trigger the starvation system in your body. Not eating causes the blood sugar to decrease and will stimulate fat storing hormones. The main hormone that will be released due to stress is cortisol, which can turn the muscles that you need to burn fuel and fat into sugar fuel. Creating these habits will store fat around your organs in the abdomen.

This cortisol response will also deplete your level of DHEA, dehydroepiandrosterone, which is needed to create a stabilizing effect on all body systems, including converting calories to heat instead of being stored as fat. DHEA helps the body to build lean muscle tissue which helps with fighting fat in and on your body. Eating something every two to three hours will have a profound effect on your metabolism and will decrease the stress on the body's hormones.

2. *Sugar, Grains and Fats.* Avoid eating refined sugars and refined grains, which affect fat burning more than eating actual fats. Eating sugar-based foods will trigger the most powerful fat making and storing hormone--Insulin. When insulin is increased it will block fat from being used as fuel and convert sugar to fat. High fructose corn syrup is in almost every boxed, bagged, or canned food we buy, and will cause weight gain.

In Science Daily, March 22nd 2010, a Princeton University research team demonstrated that this was true. Participants who consumed high fructose corn syrup gained more weight compared to those who ate normal table sugar, even when the overall calorie intake was the same. In addition to causing significant weight gain, long term consumption of high fructose corn syrup also led to abnormal increases in body fat, especially in the abdomen. This also increased a rise in blood fats called triglycerides. When you buy foods from a grocery store, look at the labels and ingredients to see if this toxin is present. If you see high fructose corn syrup in the label, decide if you're trying to put weight on or take it off.

Grains. For thousands of years the grains humans ate came straight from the stock. It was full of fiber, healthy fats, vitamins, minerals, plant enzymes, hormones and hundreds of other phyto-chemicals. Even when learning how to grind grain we received all of the richness that grains pack in their three layers. Whole grains have a tough fibrous outer layer called bran that protects the inside of the kernel. The interior part contains mostly the starchy endosperm. Its job is to provide stored energy for the germ, the seed's reproductive kernel.

The germ is rich in vitamins, minerals and unsaturated oils. The invention of the roller mills in the late 19th century changed what we got from grains. Milling strips away the bran and germ, making the grain easier to chew, easier to digest, and easier to keep without refrigeration. The healthy oils in the germ can turn rancid causing a bad taste. Milling and processing pulverizes the endosperm from a small solid nugget into millions of particles. Refining whole wheat grain creates fluffy flour that makes light airy breads and pastries. This process destroys the wholesome nutrition that is in the grain. This process can strip away more than half of the wheat's B vitamins, 90% of the vitamin E and almost all of the fiber; not to mention the pesticides and insecticides it leaves behind; and the preservatives that create a long shelf life.

This processing will affect the balance of hormones and cause up regulation and mimic estrogen and cause endocrine hormone disruption. This also contributes to the difficulty some people have today in losing weight.

Fats are essential for the function of our bodies. They are neutral and have little effect on fat storing hormones. In the 1960s we were told to eat a low fat, low cholesterol diet to lose weight and prevent or control heart disease and other chronic conditions. We then saw fat free or foods touted as lower in fat springing up all over the grocery stores.

Overall, this has not helped us with the weight loss battle. Americans taking this advice and eating lower fat foods have not seen the results in weight loss as a result of less fat in their diet. In fact, in the 1960s 13% of the population was obese compared to 34% today; and only 1% had type II diabetes, compared to 8% today. Actually, the total amount of fat in the diet isn't really linked with weight or disease according to Harvard (Howard BV, Manson JE, Stefanick ML ET AL. Low fat dietary pattern and weight change over seven years, Women's Health Initiative, Dietary Modification trial, Jama 2006; 295-39-49).

So what are good fats? The answer is unsaturated fat. Unsaturated fats are called "good" because they can improve blood cholesterol levels, ease inflammation, and help heart rhythms, along with other benefits. These fats are found in foods from plants, nuts and seeds. Two types of unsaturated fats are monounsaturated fats, which come from eating raw nuts and seeds, olive oil, avocado, almonds, hazelnuts, pecans and pumpkin and sesame seeds. The other unsaturated fat is polyunsaturated fats, which include Omega 3s, fat which the body cannot make. These must come from food--fish and plant sources, chia seeds, flax seeds and walnuts.

Our bodies can make all the saturated fats we need. We don't need to consume much of this fat. Too much saturated fat will cause weight gain, not to mention cardiovascular disease. Eating meat, seafood, poultry with skin, dairy products, cheese, milk and ice cream, plants with coconut oil or palm oil should be kept to a minimum in your diet.

Bad Fats or transfats are made by heating liquid vegetable oils in the presence of hydrogen gas called hydrogenation. Partially hydrogenating vegetable oils makes them more stable and gives them a longer shelf life. Partially hydrogenated oils can withstand repeated heating, such as in frying fast foods and in restaurants. These foods have a damaging effect on the body, not to mention the inflammation it causes.

Commercially prepared baked goods, margarine, snack foods, processed foods, French fries and other fried foods contain these fats. Trans fats fire up the inflammation of the body and affect the immune system, as well as affecting all other degenerative conditions that cause disease such as heart attacks, strokes, obesity, diabetes, joint pain and other chronic conditions in our bones as well. Eliminating Tran's fats from our food supply could prevent 6-20% of diseases, totaling 200,000 per year.

3.   *Emotional Eating.* Overeating and emotional eating is also something you should try to avoid. Emotional eating is the practice of consuming large quantities of food, usually comfort or junk foods due to emotional feelings rather than hunger. Experts claim that 75% of overeating is caused by emotions. Many people learn growing up that food can bring comfort. We turn to food to heal emotional problems because it changes our physiological state. Any kind of situation we do not like to be in, we escape by eating (or smoking, drinking or taking drugs) that change our physiological state to a happier one.

Depression, boredom, loneliness, chronic anger, anxiety, frustration, stress, problems with relationships, and self-esteem issues all can result in overeating and weight gain. This trend of overeating will cause stress to the body, which causes the adrenals to release cortisol and decreases DHEA, increases blood sugar levels, increases insulin, increases fat storing hormones and not the fat burning ones you're trying to trigger.

How can you break yourself of the habit of emotional eating? First, identify eating triggers to help alter the emotional eating. Then develop alternatives to eating such as reading a good book or magazine or listening to music; going for a walk or jog; taking a bubble bath; doing deep breathing exercises; playing cards or games; talking to a friend; doing housework, yard work or laundry; washing the car;

writing a letter or any other pleasurable activity you enjoy that will decrease the urge to eat. These distractions will help to reprogram your thoughts and change your emotions towards food.

Another tool we use at Club Reduce is SMT, self-mastery technology. This is done to change how you think about and react towards food. What if a person could completely change their lives using relaxation? What if rewiring the brain to implement weight loss into one's life was as simple as putting on headphones to listen to music and vocal help, adding sunglasses with flickering light at a certain speed to change the subconscious to the conscious forever and live without ever feeling the need to overeat again? With SMT we make it possible.

4. *Alcohol.* Avoid consuming alcohol. Alcohol triggers insulin and causes weight gain. Alcohol can cause liver damage which stresses the body to produce more cortisol and depletes DHEA levels. Alcohol can reduce fat burning by a third. This is not good for those of you trying to lose weight and get your body into fat burning mode. If you booze you don't lose. When you drink alcohol it's broken down into acetate, which is basically vinegar, which will be burned up before any of the food calories are used from eating or from what is stored on your body.

By giving your body all its energy from the acetate you consumed as alcohol, you're left with potential energy stores as fat on your tummy and hips. Alcohol temporarily inhibits lipid oxidation. In other words, when alcohol is in your system it's harder for your body to burn the fat that's already there. Alcohol will stretch your body's systems in the cortisol chain of events and increases your love handles. This is not going to get your fat burning hormones kicked up.

5. *Caffeine.* Consuming caffeine and drinking coffee or colas can play havoc. If you drink caffeinated beverages throughout the day you may actually be causing yourself to eat more. If you struggle to lose weight you may want to kick this habit. Caffeine intake will increase your snacking throughout the day and you'll eat even more for lunch.

Decreasing caffeine can and will help control food cravings. How does this craving of foods start? Caffeine raises the stress hormone cortisol. Cortisol raises the heart rate, increases the blood sugar, and signals your body to increase energy stores. This increases your want for something sweet and sugary. This is evident after lunch, in the early afternoon when the cravings for sweet foods hit and you're down at the vending machines at work. This could be due to the morning coffee you had for breakfast.

Caffeine can trigger hypoglycemia which can trigger appetite and cravings for higher calorie foods. The more caffeine consumed, the more you want to eat. Caffeine can make you feel jittery and affect your physical, mental and emotional wellbeing. Caffeine induced stress can affect how you feel about yourself and trigger emotional eating or comfort food, not to mention overeating causing weight gain. Caffeine can lead to feelings of depression.

As mentioned before caffeine increases cortisol levels and with prolonged raised levels can:

- lower your immune system
- slow your thinking
- blood sugar imbalances
- Increase fat making hormones
- increase blood pressure
- weaken muscles
- Weakens bones, causing osteoporosis.
- increase fat in the stomach, tummy areas, belly fat

Caffeine has shown to contribute to insulin resistance. When this happens, insulin and glucose build up in the blood. Coffee can also cause insomnia and sleep deprivation. There are a lot of symptoms and diseases that are caused by increased levels of insulin than insulin resistance, other than weight gain.

Club Reduce offers a replacement for your coffee. It will give you energy and necessary vitamins, enzymes, minerals, amino acids, essential protein that caffeine drinks cannot do for you. Call the office for your free sample, which comes in chocolate, strawberry, vanilla and orange cream.

6.   *Exercise -- When and how and how much? Anaerobic versus aerobic.* The term aerobic exercise means you are causing the body to utilize oxygen to create energy. The oxygen is needed to break down glucose. Glucose is the fuel needed to create energy. Anaerobic is the opposite of aerobic in that it creates energy without oxygen. The body's demand for energy is greater, so it finds natural body chemicals to fuel it. To determine whether you are doing aerobic or anaerobic exercise is to monitor your heart rate while exercising. For men, the maximum heart rate is 220 less your age. For women it is 225 less your age.

The goal rate for exercising should be 70% of your maximum rate. When your heart rate reaches over 70% you are doing aerobic exercise. Any movement your body makes requires energy. You don't have to do just aerobic exercise to lose weight or maintain a desired weight. Aerobic exercise has more of an impact on the cardiovascular and circulatory systems.

I have patients that walk every day on a treadmill or outside and cannot lose weight. Light to moderate aerobic exercise can help start you off on a weight loss course. This type of exercise includes classes, treadmills, exercise bikes, ski machines, air gliders, jogging. When you start the day with aerobic exercise you will burn glucose for the first fifteen to twenty five minutes before any fat is used up. Aerobic exercise will burn 25% muscle and 75% fat only while you're exercising. Once you stop exercising the fat burning stops.

Most people think all they need to do is exercise to lose weight. The truth is your body may not be healthy enough to exercise. When your body is not balanced in the area of digestion and the elimination of toxins you can put additional stress on your body. Additional stress to your body affects the adrenals, which in the case of negative stress will release cortisol. Remember, cortisol is a fat making hormone. This is why you need to consult a doctor that understands the different levels of exercise to see if you're healthy enough to start an exercise program.

Don't get down on yourself because you go to the gym every day and see nothing change on your body. Most people that go to the gym are on the cardio machines. Very few are hitting the weights. Why would lifting weight help you to lose more weight? First of all, we all know how to walk. That's why you see more people in the gym performing activities they know how to do. The weights and weight machines may look intimidating to say the least. What if I do it wrong? I don't want anybody to see me over there because I might look stupid. That's why gyms have trainers to help you on the weight machines until you feel comfortable with them.

It has been said that performing anaerobic exercise like weight lifting, using machines that offer resistance, and dumbbells can burn more calories on a ratio of five to one--even as much as seven to one has been reported. This type of exercise burns up to 100% fat in the body. This type of exercise will also help to produce more lean muscle mass which decreases body fat. The great thing about performing anaerobic exercise is that when you're done you're still burning fat 24-48 hours later.

To successfully benefit from anaerobic exercise you need to have healthy adrenal glands. If you do too much anaerobic with a weakened adrenal gland you can stop fat burning. Recovering after working out is vital to your success. Here at Club Reduce we can check to see if your adrenals are able to handle any workout or to see why you have not benefited from your current workouts. We also have a supplement that can help to support the adrenals.

7. *Stress and Weight Gain--How Stress Can Affect your Weight.*
Stress comes in different stages in life, along with emotional, physical and chemical stressors. All these types of stressors that we become exposed to can contribute to weight gain. When stress reaches above comfort levels the fat storing hormone called cortisol is released. Cor-

tisol comes from the adrenal glands. If you let this extra stress get to you for prolonged periods of time, called chronic stress, your health becomes at risk. This will cause weight gain and a host of other health problems. Chronic stress and cortisol can cause weight gain in the following ways.

*Metabolism-too much cortisol can slow down metabolism causing more weight gain than you normally will have on your body. This happens even if you are eating the same amount of food you have always eaten.

*Cravings--when you're really stressed you tend to crave more fatty, salt and sugary foods. The adrenal gland loves saturated fats when stressed. Salt is also craved and used in the adrenal gland. When prolonged periods of stress are experienced and cortisol levels are higher, the body increases blood sugar, which increases insulin, a fat making hormone. Once these blood sugars are used following a stressful event, the body craves sugar to maintain function of all organs and nerves.

*Elevated Blood Sugar--elevated blood sugar levels can cause mood swings, fatigue and can lead to hyperglycemia, which is elevated blood sugar levels above 140. With prolonged blood sugar levels causes inflammation in the blood vessels causing heart attacks and leading to diabetes.

*Fat Storage--excess stress affects how we store fat on our bodies. When stress levels become higher for prolonged periods of time, fat develops along the abdomen leading to increased visceral fat. The visceral fat is below the belly muscle and can cause greater health risks than if it was stored elsewhere on your body. With stress in our lives we tend to take shortcuts to decrease our stress like eating fast foods due to the time needed to plan or cook healthy foods. This can lead to emotional eating.

When we need to change our current feelings to be happy, we eat. This changes our physiological state, which means it takes us from felling stressed to happy. We want to be in a different state and have different feelings from where we are now. This is why so many people have bad habits. They are trying to change from one state of feeling to become happy and feel good now. This can happen with food. We have no time to exercise. This only stresses us more. Studies have actually shown that exercise can lessen stress on our bodies. Exercise is a natural way to decrease stress and how we feel it and deal with it.

When we are stressed DHEA levels are depleted causing weight gain. We need to feel good right now no matter what comes our way. Learn to deal with stress. Take time for yourself, get up a little earlier to organize yourself, plan your day, week and year. Being more organized has shown to lessen life stressors.

We carry natural herbs from Solutions4 to help combat stress and how our bodies deal with it.

8. *Sleep and Weight Gain.* Weight gain is one of the side effects of lack of sleep. Several studies have shown that this is the case. In the journal Sleep, 2010, 35,000 employees of an electric power company were studied. Most employees were male. The study found that men who slept five or less hours a night were more likely to experience weight gain than those who slept seven to eight hours a night. Too much sleep, nine plus hours, also showed to gain weight in these men.

Women are also affected according to a 2006 study from the Case Western Reserve University in Cleveland. Women who slept less than five hours a night were 32% more likely to gain 33 pounds or more per year over a sixteen year study than women who slept at least seven hours a night.

Lack of sleep lowers the leptin levels. Leptin is a protein that regulates and controls appetite. Low levels of leptin may increase appetite which can lead to eating more and causing weight gain. This can also lead to sleep apnea due to gaining weight in the throat and decreasing the breathing pathway. Obesity causes sleep apnea, which leads to more weight gain.

The trick is to get to bed between 9:00 to 10:00 p.m. Retiring to bed earlier will allow you to reach the deep REM, rapid eye movement, sleep. By midnight growth hormone is released for up to two hours. Growth hormone is a fat burning hormone. This is why not only sleeping seven to eight hours is good but it's important to sleep throughout the night without getting up to use the bathroom. Getting up in the night to urinate could be a sign of pre diabetes, Candida, or prostate swelling in men.

Some suggestions for going to bed at a good time: Take a warm bath, read a good book--not a really good book because you may not want to put it down--read something uplifting, positive and motivating such as self-help books. Avoid watching TV due to all the negative news. Spend time in the evening with family and friends and avoid eating later than 6-7:00 p.m. Decrease your water intake after 6 o'clock at night.

9. *Protein and Weight Loss.* There are a lot of weight loss diets that recommend protein to help lose weight. There is a low protein diet. There is a high protein diet and the even higher protein diet. How much protein do we really need? Which is best? What foods contain it? Does exercising more create more need for protein? It is true that protein at the right levels and from the right source can trigger fat burning hormones such as glucagon and growth hormone. The more active you are the more protein you need.

What is protein? Protein is made up of twenty building blocks called amino acids. Of those twenty the body makes eleven nonessential amino acids. The other nine are called essential amino acids and must be supplied by what we eat. There are two kinds of dietary proteins, complete and incomplete. Animal and soy proteins are complete because they contain all nine essential amino acids. Plants like vegetables, nuts, fruits and legumes are incomplete because they lack one or more essential amino acid. This is why if you plan to get your protein (amino acids) from plants, you need to eat a variety of these foods.

Protein can help to curb your appetite which helps with weight loss. Protein plays an important role in our bodies. Proteins provide essential building blocks to repair the cells that die and slough off of our hair, bones, skin, vital organs and any function of the body. Protein at the right levels and balance can help regulate sleep and support hormones.

For all these functions the body needs complete proteins. Our body can also receive the protein it needs by eating a variety of plant products throughout the day. These can supply our needs without eating animal or soy products. Eating a combination of plant proteins and amino acids will provide the body with the essential nutrients to build the protein needed for growth and function. Protein is, again, a branch chain of amino acids which have to be broken down in the stomach before they can be assimilated into the body.

It takes a lot of energy to break the protein amino acid bonds. Plant foods supply the amino acids already broken down, and are much more easily assimilated into the blood to be used to repair the cells and also to help with function. The amount of protein one needs varies with the activity of that person during the day. By eating more plant based proteins we avoid what the animal proteins come with. Animal proteins are full of hormones. They help the animal grow larger, lay more eggs. Antibiotics are used to keep the animal from dying due to the closeness of the population they are raised in.

When we eat the animal that has been injected with antibiotics, we are in a sense ingesting; taking in the drug which is like always being on the drug. This will kill the good bacteria that are there to help in the digesting of food. When healthy bacteria are killed off, yeast can grow and spread throughout the body causing many symptoms including weight gain. There are a lot of problems with yeast over growth. This was covered in chapter four. Commercial animal proteins are high in fat due to the inactivity of the animal.

The animal based proteins that are the easiest and less stressful to digest would be fish and then chicken. The other meats, beef, pork, and other four legged animals are very acidic and cause inflammation and joint damage may occur. There are many alternatives to eating animal proteins--such as whey. The Solutions4 products that we carry in our office are lactose and dairy free and the whey in the meal replacement shake tastes amazing.

How much protein do we need? The RDA recommends 0.4 grams per pound of ideal body weight. Note: ideal body weight is where you should be, not necessarily what you weigh now. To figure out the protein grams you need simply multiply your weight by 0.4. For a person that weighs 200 pounds that's 80 grams. That's four small cans of tuna fish per day. For a 170 pound man it would equal 68 grams. For a woman weighing 135 pounds, that is 54 grams of protein. The more active you are during the day including exercise may require more protein, from 0.6 to 0.7 grams multiplied by your ideal body weight. This can include more dense green foods and supplementing your diet with the Solutions4 shake to fulfill your needs if you want to avoid animal products.

QUICK WEIGHT LOSS TIP:

One of the quickest ways to increase weight loss is to do a detoxification cleansing and elimination program. We have a detoxification kit that will last from three to ten days for purification, improving digestive function especially proteins, and strengthening vital organs. Call Club Reduce to get your kit to start your weight loss program off successfully.

C H A P T E R
N I N E

*Unlocking Your Health
At The Speed of Thought*

Unlocking Your Health
At The Speed of Thought

Achieving your life and health goals can be as easy as taking a breath in open air. The trick is in learning how to use your mind to get what you want.

Whether you realize it or not, at every moment you are affirming something for your life. When it comes to your body, you are either affirming health or you are affirming illness. Which tells us that healing starts with a thought.

An American Indian elder once described his own internal struggles this way: "Inside of me there are two dogs. One of the dogs is mean and evil. The other dog is good. The mean dog fights the good dog all the time." When asked which dog wins, he reflected for a moment and replied, "The one I feed the most."

We use this elder's story as a metaphor about how our minds work. When you give thoughts energy, or when you feed them with emotion, they will grow. This is true whether the thought is good or bad, harmful or helpful. The purpose of this chapter is to teach you how to feed the right dog—the healthy dog. Using positive affirmations does all this.

What is a Self-Mastery Affirmation?

An affirmation is a specific statement that elicits a response. Affirmations can be either spoken or written. For maximum benefit, they should always be stated in the positive. Affirmative declarations, when stated consistently, help you visualize and realize your goals. By affirming what you want each day, you are doing something positive toward fulfilling your dream of losing weight and keeping it off.

It has been said that a picture is worth a thousand words. If this is so, how does a spoken or written word change your self-image?

Well, that's where Self-Mastery Affirmations come in. We train you to use specific language patterns that create the mental pictures you want. By using positive affirmations, you are the producer and director of your inner theater; you are directing your mind to create what you want. In other words, you become the "Steven Spielberg" of your mind!

People tend to use a great deal of thought power on what they don't want instead of what they do want. Unfortunately, your mind tends to give you exactly what you dwell on, which, in this instance, is what you don't want.

As an example, imagine that you are a business owner and have just hired a new assistant. You spend the entire first morning training your new assistant on everything you don't want her to do. When you are finished, you leave for lunch.

What is your assistant going to do?

You guessed it, everything you don't want her to do. After all, what choice does she have when you never told her what you want? Another answer may be: Nothing at all. Again, she doesn't know what to do!

I once counseled a middle-aged man named Tony who desperately wanted to beat his buddies on the golf course. The only problem was, no matter how hard he practiced, his game seemed to stay the same or worsen. He sat in the chair across from me and frowned. "I practice and practice but nothing happens."

This was the opening I was looking for. "What did you just say," I asked.

"I practice and practice and nothing happens," Tony repeated.

"Then you're getting exactly what you ask for," I said.

Tony stared at me with unblinking eyes. "What do you mean," he asked. "That's not what I want."

"I know," I said, "that's why you're here. Unfortunately, you've been practicing affirmations without the proper training."

Tony's eyebrows shot up.

"The way you speak to yourself has powerful implications," I said. "That's why Henry Ford said, 'Whether you think you can or think you can't, you are right!' The same is true with your golf game. Whether you think you will improve or not improve, you are right. What would you prefer happen with your golf game?" I took out an index card and handed it to Tony. "I mean if your wildest dreams could come true?"

"I would break ninety consistently," he answered.

"So, would an affirmation like, I am scoring at an 89 or lower, make sense?"

"Yes, I think that would work." Tony replied.

"Then go ahead and write it down in your own words. Just make sure it's stated in the positive."

After Tony had written his affirmation, I asked him to place the card in his pocket. "Whenever you notice an unwanted thought about your golf swing," I said, "just stop yourself and then take out the index card and read it. Better yet, when you hear the inner negative thought, say to yourself, backspace/delete, and then take out the card and read it. Read it out load whenever possible."

Tony looked pensive for moment. He then touched the pocket with the affirmation card tucked inside and smiled.

"See," I said, "it's working already."

His smile broadened.

"This is only one piece of the puzzle," I reminded him, "and it takes practice. Your mind operates through your senses and they all play a roll."

For Tony this was significant in relation to his golf game, but he also found that the habit of affirming his goals and desires had a positive effect in many other aspects of his life.

So what about you? What words do you regularly say to yourself in regard to your body or weight? What pictures do these words create in your mind? What emotions arise? Let's take a moment to determine what kind of self-talk you have going that might be limiting your ability to lose weight.

Do you have any of these negative affirmations scripting your life?

If you can answer yes to any of the following statements, Self-Mastery Affirmations are your key to re-scripting your life.

1.   Do you make negative statements or have negative beliefs about yourself that you repeat internally throughout the day?

2.   Do you use negative statements about yourself in your every¬day conversations with family, friends or coworkers?

3.   Do self-deprecating remarks negatively influence your behavior, such as causing you to procrastinate?

4.   Do you still believe the negative comments made by members

of your family or friends when you were young?

5. Do you replay negative feedback you get from your spouse, boss, teacher, colleagues, children, parents, and relatives? Does this get in the way of achieving your goals?

6. Do you have a negative self-image of any part of your body that you visualize, and then allow it to influence how you present yourself to others?

7. Do you have negative self-talk based on assessments others have made of your competency, skills, ability, knowledge, intelligence, creativity, or common sense?

8. Do you have negative stories about your past behavior, failures, or performances that you systematically run through your mind and that influence your current conduct?

9. Do you have a negative attitude about your potential for achievement? Does this attitude influence your motivation, stop your effort, and kill your drive?

10. Do you have feelings of guilt, either real or imagined, that prevent positive inner thoughts?

11. Do you discuss negative prophecies that you or others have made about your future, your success, your relationships, your family, or your health; do these haunt you as you face a daily struggle to "win" at weight loss or at the game of life?

12. Do you use negative visualization or self-talk to your personal detriment?

How do you change these internal messages?

Your best thinking brought you to this very moment. If you aren't getting what you want, then you will need to upgrade your thinking. Unfortunately, you can't go to the corner software store and purchase the latest upgrade. But don't worry; we'll work together through Self-Mastery Technology to turn you into your own software engineer for your mind.

The first step in programming is to know the language you are using; in our case, we'll be using the language of the mind.
What we say and what the mind hears can be completely different. For instance, let's imagine we are at a family function and little Jimmy is

running toward the door. Someone yells, "Don't slam the door!" Jimmy runs out and...SLAM! The next thing you know poor Jimmy is sitting in the corner in time out. Jimmy has no idea why he's being punished. In his mind, he did exactly what he was told to do. You see, the subconscious mind doesn't know how to process a negative. When Jimmy heard, "Don't slam the door," his mind created a picture of him slamming the door.

Here's a great example. If I ask you not to think about dancing pink elephants, what happens?
You can't help but think about them, right?

To be a software engineer for the mind is to eliminate negative thoughts and replace them with statements that are affirming. This seems simple enough on the surface, but putting it into practice is another matter. This is where the Self-Mastery Technology comes in. A good engineer will have a proto-type, which is a working model, but not a production model. If the proto-type works, it will then go into production.

The affirmations you will create here should be thought of as proto-types; if they work in the laboratory of your mind, you will then put them into production in your life.

Now here are Some Tips for Writing Self-Mastery Affirmations

Always state what you want in the first person (I or I am). State your affirmation in the positive and as if it is occurring or has already occurred.

Examples:
"I am living a slim lifestyle one day at a time."
"I am enjoying my body at 145 lbs or less."
"I am drinking health-giving water daily."
"I am a healthy person."
"I am excited to be at my ideal weight."
...and so forth.

Now give your affirmation energy. Empower it with emotion.

Imagine yourself fulfilling the affirmation. See it in full living color, hear the sounds, and imagine how you feel while living the affirmation. In other words, engage all your senses.

Let's use the following affirmation: "I look great at parties and easily say no to Candida-causing foods."
When you read the affirmation, are you picturing your shoulders rolled back? Is your head high?

What are other factors that would convince you that the affirmation is true for you? What are you hearing? What happens when your favorite music is in the background? There are no limits in the imagination, so feel free to dream up precisely the life you want.
Be sure to write all affirmations in your own handwriting. Read the affirmations aloud, with emotion, at least once a day so you can be reminded of their intrinsic value.

Most people have spent the greater part of their lives telling themselves what not to do and we all know that doesn't work! Your mind is starving for the loving tone of your own voice reinforcing positive thoughts and patterns.

In my book, Awaken the Genius, Mind Technology for the 21st Century, I have a section about affirmations and how they work. We go deeper into this area by discussing what I describe in my book as impact words.

So Just What is an Impact Word?

An impact word is a word or series of words that has a direct impact on you. As an example, if learning were important to you in the context of your job, you would be drawn toward employment ads that use the term learning in its description. As an example: Seeking intelligent, resourceful person to help develop weight-loss programs. Must be willing to learn and apply new knowledge to help clients get noticeable results.

Impact words also house our values or trigger our value system when they are used. These words help run meta-programs, or the programs of the subconscious.

How can these words be of benefit to you?

First, if you know what these words are, you can use them to create more powerful affirmations and more beneficial behaviors. Continuing with the example of learning, if you use that word in you're Self-Mastery Affirmation, it will have more impact. Example: "I enjoy learning and applying information about a healthy lifestyle."

Second, you can find out how these words are giving energy to unwanted behaviors. Let's use the example of the word, challenge, which is a somewhat common impact word. Many of the clients I see will tell me they enjoy a good challenge. If they are having trouble losing weight and "challenge" is one of their impact words, the excitement of the "challenge" inherent in losing, or not losing, weight may be working against them, and may override the benefits of being naturally thin. The person might even have a negative response to the word 'thin," because they feel they were passed by when the "thin" genes were handed out. They can look at a thin person and get angry without knowing why. In this case, desire for a challenge and the goal of being thin are in conflict and the person will not lose weight. To correct this habit, an effective affirmation might be, "I enjoy the challenge of thinking and eating like a healthy person."

Now let's discover your impact words so you can get started putting them to work for you.

At the top of a blank sheet of paper write down the word "Job." What has to be present in a job for you to enjoy it? Write down the answers that come into your mind. Some past clients gave answers like:

1. a challenge
2. freedom to do it my way
3. flexible hours
4. a stimulating environment
5. working with people
6. variety in what I'm doing

Next write down the word "Relationship." What has to be present in a relationship for you to enjoy it? Examples I have heard in the past are:

1. There has to be communication
2. Closeness or a physical attraction
3. Common purpose or goals
4. The person has to be fun loving
5. He or she has to be intelligent
6. The person must be into a healthy lifestyle

Next write down a "Hobby" that you enjoy. What is present in that hobby that causes you to enjoy it? Clients have responded with statements like:

1. Its a distraction
2. Its a challenge
3. Its fun
4. Its stimulating
5. It gets me out of the house
6. It's a creative outlet

Next write down how you know that you have done a good job? You have two choices here. You know when someone else tells you. As an example, Frank just finishes painting the living room. He is unsure if he has done a good job. Then the moment of truth. His wife walks in. She is thrilled with the job Frank did. She comments on how good it looks. At that moment Frank knows the job is right. He feels it inside. He knows when something external, someone else or something else, tells him.

Let's imagine that George paints his living room. He is sure it's done well. He cleans up the brushes and puts away the paint. His wife comes in. She notices a few flaws in the job George did. George then spends several hours convincing his wife that he intended to do the painting that way. George knows he has done a good job internally.

In the area of self-help, having an internal convincer is best because this person is usually internally motivated as well. It should be noted, however, that even the most internal people I know still enjoy a hearty pat on the back for a job well done from time to time.

Now all you need are the four simple steps for putting your impact words into Self-Mastery Affirmations.

Step 1:   Let's look at creating a Self-Mastery Affirmation to take action. Using the list of words you wrote earlier, let's imagine you want to start an exercise program. You would add the impact words that motivate you into the affirmation, which empowers the mind to take action. In other words, the meta-program that runs the challenge program or the freedom program now works for your new outcome of exercising.

Sample affirmations would be:

• "I am enjoying the challenge of exercising daily." The impact words her are enjoying and challenge.
• "I am free to exercise in a way I enjoy daily." The impact words are free and enjoy.
• "I am flexible with the exercise I do daily." The impact word is flexible.
• "I am enjoying stimulating my muscles and building a fat burning machine." Here, the impact word is stimulating.
• "I am enjoying a variety of workout routines." The impact word is variety.

Step 2:   When you are creating a Self-Mastery Affirmation about yourself, your self-image, or imagining yourself in a future event, you would impact this affirmation with the relationship words. Let's use the example of learning about weight-loss using the words discovered before.

Sample SELF-MASTERY Affirmations would be:

- "I am easily communicating health information read, heard, and experienced." The impact word is communicating.
- "I am allowing a closeness with new health information and I am physically drawn to learning about ways to get healthier." The impact words are closeness and physically.
- "I have a perfect recall of information. It is stored in a way that it will serve the common purpose and help me accomplish my goals." The impact words are common purpose.
- "I am experiencing a genuine fun loving attitude about learning how to lose weight and keep it off." Here, the impact word is fun loving.
- "I am accepting my natural intelligence to learn how to take my weight off and keep it off." You guessed it, the impact word is intelligence.
- "I am totally enjoying a healthy lifestyle and am open to learning more." The impact word for this affirmation is healthy lifestyle.

Step 3: Let's take a look at how your hobby-related impact words might help you. Think about it for a minute, how resourceful would you feel if you approached your problems as if they were your hobbies? Well, if you were like my brother-in law, you would spend all your extra time, energy, and money on it. Let me explain . . .

One crisp fall morning, while the world was still engulfed in darkness, my wife Cynthia and I slept on my sisters pull out bed in her living room. We had been forewarned that the boys would be up early to go hunting. Not being hunters, we were completely unprepared for what we witnessed upon awakening.

First, my sister's husband, Russ, walked by dressed in camouflage from head to toe. He had the Rambo look down pat, right down to the bowie knife clipped to his belt. Then came Mikey. He too was in camouflage with a smaller version of the bowie knife at his side.

"Paul, let's go!" Russ yelled from the back door.

Paul, who was seven years old at the time, burst from his bedroom in full hunter garb. He ran through the room, hooking his child-sized bowie knife to his belt.

That afternoon, the fearless hunters returned empty handed.

My wife and I observed this same ritual for three straight mornings, and each day they returned with nothing. My curiosity grew stronger each day. "Russ, what do you get out of this exercise?" I asked.

I love the time with the boys," he said. "And being in nature? There's nothing else like it. Out there, I have time to think . . . and dream. It's just a great break from the daily grind."

Once Russ explained his hobby, it made perfect sense. Before that, I simply couldn't fathom his fascination with getting up at five am to go sit in the cold Michigan woods. But then again, it wasn't my hobby.

I enjoy golfing. I may even be a little obsessed with it—which is true for most golfers. Russ, on the other hand, tells me it is a game for fools. "How else could you get someone to pay $100 to run around a cow field chasing a little white ball? He says.

I spent a great deal of time explaining the intricacies of golf to him. I detailed the reasons I loved the game. I described the excitement of the challenge. I spoke passionately of how the game required a certain level of intelligence to choose the right club, and to know how to swing for every ball position.

"Give me a rifle anytime," was his reply.

At first his answer frustrated me. How could he not understand the thrill in golf? But then I remembered, it wasn't his hobby.

Think about your hobby. How much time, energy, and money have you spent on it this year? What would happen if you put that same kind of motivation into changing something about yourself?

For this exercise, let's focus on your goal to lose weight. Sample suggestions would be:

- "I am enjoying my healthy eating distraction." Can you guess the impact words here? That's right, enjoying and distraction.
- "I am enjoying my challenge of weighing 145 or less." How about here? If you said challenge, you are correct.
- "I am having more fun eating healthy than I thought possible." Did you recognize fun as the impact word here?
- "I am stimulating my metabolic rate by drinking 8-10 glasses

of water." This one might be a little tricky. If you guessed stimulating, you are correct.

• "I am experimenting with a healthy lifestyle that is getting me out of the house." Do you remember this one? The impact words here involve getting out of the house.

• "I am allowing a creative solution to my weight problem of the past." Of course, the impact word here is creative.

Step 4: Now it is time to apply the knowledge of your convincer. Remember, this relates to the question, "How do you know if you've done a good job." If someone or something outside of you must tell you, then your convincer is external. If you know inside, then your convincer is internal.

The other-than-conscious mind works best when you start with the end in mind. What we know about the convincer is that it will work even quicker and easier if we pace your belief about the outcome.

Let's imagine that you want to exercise more regularly. An example Self-Mastery Affirmation for the externally convinced would be:

• "I am enjoying the praise from my friends and family as I exercise 4 times a week."

An internally convinced sample would be:

• "I am enjoying the quiet confidence I feel after an exercise session."

Do you see the difference? The secret to using the hobby impact word list is using it directly in your Self-Mastery Affirmations. They key is in taking the time to imagine the days, weeks and months to come. This is where you can use your Self-Mastery Affirmations to optimum advantage.

Now it's time for you to write your own Self-Mastery

Affirmations. For example, if you had creativity as an impact word it could be used in an affirmation such as: "I am creatively improving my body one day at a time."

If the impact word was happiness then the affirmation could be: "I am happily drinking water to stimulate my body to be a fat burning machine." If the impact word was freedom then it could be: "I am freeing my mind to learn at an accelerated rate."

Now Take a Few Minutes to Do Your SELF-MASTERY Affirmation Exercise

There's no time like the present to create your own Self-Mastery Affirmations.

I have given you a great start by creating some affirmations for you. Each includes some typical impact words. Read through all the sample affirmations and circle the impact word that has greatest significance for you. If you have an impact word that's not listed, but that would have greater meaning for you, write it in the blank.

After you've completed all ten, choose the affirmation that has the most meaning to you. This is the affirmation you will use this week. Next week choose another affirmation, and then another the following week, and so on. After that, you can create your own affirmations or use any of the ten examples again. When you have determined the affirmation you want to use for the week, write it on the 3x5 card. Carry the card with you during the day and read the affirmation at least ten times a day.

Well, even though the brain and mind make up an incredibly complex system, getting it all to work for you is really quite simple, once you know how.

As you state the affirmation, imagine how you will take it with you out into the world. These affirmations can be there for you whenever a challenge or opportunity arises. Start by thinking of three places where you're going to use your affirmation. It could be when you turn on a light switch and the inner light of awareness comes on and reminds you that you are mastering life. It could happen when you turn on the ignition of your car and you ignite an affirmation to start running in your life. It could happen when you open the refrigerator door, and you remember that you are opening your mind to choices . . . and you choose to use Self-Mastery Affirmations to help you make positive changes and accomplish your loftiest goals.

Sample Affirmations

1.   I am _____ improving my body each day.
(joyfully, successfully, meaningfully, creatively, passionately)

2.   I am _____ eating less, whether dining in or out.
(enjoying, easily, successfully, effortlessly, simply)

3.   I am really proud of myself for _____ taking the time to exercise.
(successfully, easily, freely, happily, creatively)

4.   I am _____ realizing my weight-loss goals each day.
(easily, successfully, wisely, passionately, enthusiastically)

5.   I am calm, relaxed and _____ as I make healthy food choices and lose weight.
(successful, positive, creative, happy, free)

6.   I am_____ drinking water to stimulate my body to be a fat burning machine.
(easily, freely, triumphantly, confidently, joyfully)

7.   I am _____ eating only those foods which are beneficial to me.
(gladly, easily, wisely, enthusiastically, confidently)

8.   I am gaining _____ everyday as I lose weight.
(self-esteem, happiness, confidence, satisfaction, freedom)

9.   Right now and at all times I see myself as healthy, trim, and
_____.

(whole, happy, free, energized, light, successful)

10.   I find it _____ to leave food on my plate at mealtimes.
(simple, encouraging, wonderful, effortless, rewarding)

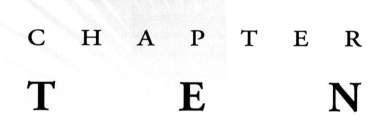

CHAPTER

T E N

Nutritional Supplements

ANTIOXIDANT

A growing body of scientific research indicates that astaxanthin has the ability to provide exceptionally powerful antioxidant protection to cells and has functional effects on muscle and nerve physiology. Comprehensive studies find astaxanthin to be ten times more effective than beta-carotene and many times more effective than vitamin E. Astaxanthin is a polyunsaturated free radical quencher and part of a series of compounds including beta-carotene included in the family of carotenoid antioxidants. These compounds add color to vegetables (red, orange, yellow) in which they occur naturally. This specific carotenoid also gives sea foods like salmon and shrimp their red coloration.

Astaxanthin nutrients are the most potent antioxidants in all of nature, and have been proven to work longer than other antioxidants in protecting against photosensitized oxidation. It has been shown that dietary astaxanthin exerts anti-tumor activity through the enhancement of immune response.

Suggested Use: 2 capsules two times daily 2
capsules two times daily will last: 15 days
Size Available: 60 capsules
Shelf Life: 7 years

Ingredients:

ASTAXANTHIN — Has anti-inflammatory properties, stimulates the immune system, and has anti-cancer effects on human cells. Also prevents oxidative damage to blood LDL-cholesterol.

ANGEL HAIR (MOZUKU) — A Japanese sea plant that promotes healthy living and helps the body to fight disease.

GINKGO BILOBA — Helps ease digestive problems and stomach complaints.

BILBERRY FRUIT — Acts as an antioxidant that purifies the blood and can be used as a diuretic.

MILK THISTLE HERB — Helps relieve the symptoms of hepatitis, cirrhosis, and inflammatory liver conditions. It is one of the most effective herbs known for relieving liver disorders.

SELENIUM CHELATE — An important mineral with potent antioxidant properties. Is important for protecting cells from the damaging effects of free radicals.

MOTHERWORT — A digestive bitter and as such encourages bile production, healthy digestion and reduces gas pains.

GREEN TEA EXTRACT — Inhibits fat-digesting lipase enzymes of the stomach and pancreas.

RED RASPBERRY EXTRACT — A blood tonic.

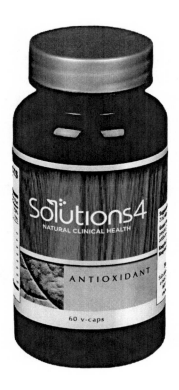

APPETITE APPEASER

A natural formulation developed to balance blood sugar levels in the body, helping to appease the appetite and increase energy levels. Helps to reduce nervous tension, eliminate hunger pains and support the body's cleansing system. Promotes the metabolism of dangerous fat deposits that adhere to the heart and other vital organs. Solutions4 APPETITE APPEASER can be used alone or as a valuable aid to weight loss and cellulite removal.

Helps the Body To:

Produce "fat burning" enzymes•
Reduce hunger pangs•
Reduce nervous tension•
Appease the appetite naturally•
Calm the nervous system naturally•
Increase energy levels naturally•
Eliminate gas & mucus from the system•
Support the body's cleansing system•
Purify the blood stream•
Breakdown and oxidize fat•

Suggested Use: 2–3 capsules 1/2 hour before each meal
3 times daily
2 capsules three times daily will last: 15 days
3 capsules three times daily will last: 10 days
Size Available: 90 capsules
Shelf Life: 7 years

Ingredients:

CHICKWEED HERB — Great value in treating blood toxicity. Particularly useful in reducing excess fat. Used to protect damaged or inflamed tissues.

BURDOCK ROOT — Increases flow of urine and acts as a diuretic. Used to treat water retention and infections of the urinary tract. Eliminates excess nervous energy.

FENNEL SEED — Relieves gas and pains in the bowels. Has a cooling affect on the bowels. Lubricates the intestines and is very healing.

HAWTHORNE BERRIES — Normalizes blood pressure. An anti-spasmodic and sedative. Helps with strain for those under pressure. Good for circulation.

LICORICE ROOT — Contains substances similar to the adrenal hormones. Treats adrenal insufficiency. Has a stimulating action and helps counteract stress.

PARSLEY HERB — Useful for bladder infections. Builds energy. Helpful for difficult urination. Used to treat water retention. Used as a preventive herb.

DANDELION ROOT — Used for blood purification. Has properties to protect the stomach lining. Helps neutralize excess acids.

KELP (Norwegian) — Useful in maintaining a healthy condition and overcoming minor imbalances. Recommended for those who are weak and run down. Used in the recovery from acute ailments and in rebuilding energy for those suffering chronic diseases.

BLADDERWRACK — Works on the glandular system. A reducing aid to be used in conjunction with other herbs for weight problems.

GOTU KOLA — Considered one of the best herb tonics. Used for all ailments of the mind and nerves.

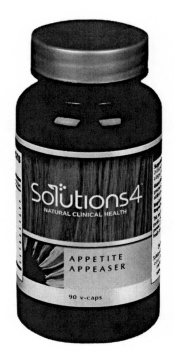

BODY PURIFIER

Solutions4 BODY PURIFIER is part of a complete Detoxification Program. This is a program that temporarily replaces a normal diet of solid food, utilizing liquid food and cleansing supplements to detoxify the body systems. The role of BODY PURIFIER in this process is to help remove toxins from the body. This supplement may also be used as an individual supplement to strengthen the immune system in times that it may be compromised.

BODY PURIFIER Helps to:

Remove congestion•
Remove mucus•
Remove environmental chemicals•
Remove harmful food additives•
Purify the blood stream•
Cleanse the lymphatic system•
Fight bacteria, virus, yeast, mold, and worms•
Restore new energy to the entire body•
Destroy parasites in the digestive system•
Suggested Use: 2–3 capsules twice daily
When utilized in a 30 — day program,
132 capsules will be used 2
capsules twice daily will last: 22 days 3
capsules twice daily will last: 15 days

Size Available: 90 capsules
Shelf Life: 7 years

An important part of the Solutions4 Detoxification program. Dosage will be adjusted accordingly when taken as a part of that program.

Ingredients:

RED CLOVER BLOSSOM — A wonderful blood purifier. Healing to new wounds as well as old ulcers. Effective in spasmodic bronchial troubles and whooping cough. Used to treat cancer because of its effects on protein assimilation.

DANDELION ROOT — Improves the function of the liver, as it has the capacity to clear obstructions while stimulating the liver to detoxify poisons. Thus, dandelion serves as a blood purifier. Also high in minerals. Useful for clearing obstructions of the spleen, pancreas, gallbladder and kidneys. Tremendous benefit to the stomach and intestines.

ECHINACEA — Echinacea is the king of blood purifiers. The most effective blood and lymphatic cleanser in the botanical kingdom. A valuable alternative to all antibiotics when used properly.

OREGON GRAPE ROOT (Barberry) — Oregon grape root stimulates the secretion of bile and thus aids in digestion and blood purification. Useful in rheumatoid arthritis, psoriasis, eczema, acne, and herpes.

QUASSIA — Tones up a run down system. Will expel worms. May destroy the appetite for strong drink.

SARSAPARILLA — Useful in the treatment of gout, rheumatism, colds, fever, ringworm, and skin eruptions, as well as other ailments requiring a good blood purifier. Will act as a powerful agent to expel gas from the stomach and intestines.

GINGER ROOT — Eliminates and counteracts the formation of mucus. Taken to relieve gas and severe pains in the bowels. Destroys parasites in the digestive system. Increases energy of the body. Stimulates circulation and breaks up obstructions.

BURDOCK ROOT AND SEED — A valuable purifier. Used in this capacity for the treatment of arthritis, rheumatism, sciatica and lumbago. Promotes kidney function and works through the kidneys to help clear the blood of harmful acids.

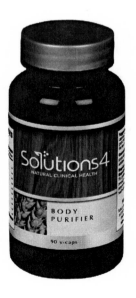

YELLOW DOCK ROOT — An astringent blood purifier useful in treating diseases of the blood and chronic skin ailments. Stimulates digestion, improving the function of the stomach and liver. Also stimulates elimination, improving flow of bile and acting as a laxative. A nutritive tonic, high in iron. Nourishes the spleen and liver. Effective for the treatment of jaundice, lymphatic problems and skin eruptions.

LIQUID CALCIUM

Unlike antacid or press tab sources of calcium, the body easily absorbs Solutions4 LIQUID CALCIUM, as it is packaged in a soluble liquid gel form. It provides the necessary 1000-2000 mg of calcium each day, and is free from yeast, corn, wheat, milk, sugar, starch, soy, preservatives, and artificial colors.

Calcium:
- *Provides strength to bones and teeth*
- *Works with magnesium for cardiovascular health*
- *Helps prevent osteoporosis*
- *Plays an important role in health, as every single cell in the body contains it.*

Calcium recommendations

Age Group	Calcium–mg
Birth–6 months	400
6 months–1 year	600
1–10 years	800–1200
11–24 years	1200–1500
25–50 years	1000
51–64 years (women on HRT & men)	1000
51–64 (women not on HRT)	1500
65 or older	1500
Pregnant or nursing	1200–1500

Suggested Use: 2–4 softgels daily 2
softgels daily will last: 50 days 4
softgels daily will last: 25 days
Size Available: 100 liquid gel capsules (500 mg each)
Shelf Life: 3 years

Ingredients:

CALCIUM CARBONATE — Helps eliminate muscle pains, cramps, twitches, and tight muscles. Lessens menstrual cramp pain, alleviates blood clotting problems, reduces nervousness and hyperactivity, helps eliminate insomnia, stops bone and teeth demineralization.

VITAMIN D — Aids in preventing colds, helps in treatment of conjunctivitis, properly utilizes calcium and phosphorous necessary for strong bones.

Additional information on natural hormone precursors indicate that Solutions4 WILD YAM CREAM, HORMONE BALANCE, and DHEA also play a role in rebuilding bone density.

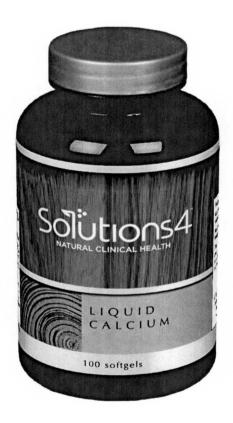

CELLULITE CLEANSE

Solutions4 CELLULITE CLEANSE contains a combination of pure, natural herbs that work together as a mild herbal diuretic to soften and break down cellulite and help stimulate and strengthen the waste elimination system. CELLULITE CLEANSE works in conjunction with the Solutions4 Detoxification program and Body Contour Wraps to increase the cleansing action of the body, preventing the formation of cellulite and assisting in its removal.

Helps the Body To:
- *Break down cellulite*
- *Eliminate waste materials as a mild, natural laxative*
- *Reduce water retention*
- *Increase body circulation*
- *Appease the appetite naturally*

When the body eliminates excess waste materials, there is nothing left to deposit in the adipose cells and connective tissue to turn to cellulite. This is an ideal condition, as most bodies are not able to eliminate excess waste that is deposited, subsequently forming cellulite. Once cellulite has formed, proper elimination is even more crucial to flush out the toxic residues. Because maximum elimination is clearly vital in solving a cellulite problem, all three organs involved — the kidneys, intestines, and the skin — must be in superb working order.

Suggested Use: Take 2-3 capsules 1/2 hour before each meal three times daily

2 capsules three times daily will last: 15 days

3 capsules three times daily will last: 10 days

Size Available: 90 capsules

Shelf Life: 7 years

Best results will be achieved when taken following a 3-day Detoxification program. Naturally, maximum results occur when this procedure is also used in conjunction with an "anti-cellulite" diet and proper exercise program.

Ingredients:

JUNIPER BERRIES — Increases the flow of urine, decreases blood pressure, and helps purify the blood. A stimulating diuretic beneficial in the treatment of urine retention, bladder discharges, and uric acid buildup.

BUCHU LEAVES — One of the best natural diuretics known. Used for all acute and chronic bladder and kidney disorders. Combined with uva ursi for the treatment of water retention and urinary tract infection.

CORN SILK — Important diuretic herb for the reduction of water in the system. One of the best remedies for kidney and bladder troubles.

HYDRANGEA ROOT — Valuable in bladder troubles. Good for chronic rheumatism. Used to release water retention.

HORSETAIL HERB — Reliable diuretic historically used for urinary disorders. This herb is rich in minerals and can aid in rebuilding new bone when used in conjunction with calcium.

UVA URSI — Aids in the treatment of bladder and kidney infections. When absorbed by the stomach, anti-microbial and astringent properties are derived. Used for vaginal infections and excessive menstruation, and to treat water retention.

KELP — Useful in maintaining overall health and balance. Recommended for those who are weak and run down. Used in the recovery of acute ailments and in rebuilding energy for those suffering chronic diseases.

LECITHIN — A key building block of cell membranes. Protects cells from oxidation and largely comprises the protective sheaths surrounding the brain. Composed mostly of B vitamins, phosphoric acid, choline, linoleic acid and inositol. A fat emulsifier that supports the circulatory system.

APPLE CIDER VINEGAR — Best known for its success in reducing body fat. Improves functioning of the body and promotes re-establishment of a normal diet. Used as a digestant.

DHEA (Dehydroepiandrosterone)

DHEA, produced in the adrenal glands, is the single-most abundant steroid in the human bloodstream. It is often called the "mother" or precursor hormone, because the body readily converts it on demand into active hormones such as estrogen, testosterone, cortisone and progesterone. DHEA declines with age more rapidly in both men and women beginning at the age of 40. This decline triggers age-related issues and increased susceptibility to disease.

Suggested Use: 1–2 capsules for women, 2–3 capsules for men 2 capsules daily will last: 45 days 3 capsules daily will last: 22 days
Size Available: 90 capsules (25mg each)
Shelf Life: 7 years

Do not use during pregnancy, while breast-feeding, or in cases of liver disease or prostate irregularity.

Ingredients:

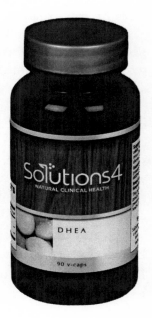

DEHYDROEPIANDROSTERONE (D.H.E.A.) — 27 mg. pure pharmaceutical grade quality per capsule. For anti-aging, hormone balance, fatigue, and immune disorders.

PIPER NIGRUM EXTRACT (BIOPERINE) — Maintains the normalcy of the digestive tract and helps in maintaining the proper peristaltic movement in the body. Helps tone the respiratory tract and urinary tract.

FIBER BLEND

Solutions4 FIBER BLEND restores dietary fiber to the system, cleans the bowels and intestines without calories, and helps to lower cholesterol levels. This specialized formula contains both soluble (Psyllium) and insoluble (Bran Powder) fiber, which work together to clean debris from the system by easing the passage of waste through the colon and absorbing toxins.

This Solutions4 formula helps to:
- *Maximize efficiency without calories*
- *Overcome constipation*
- *Cleanse bowels and intestines*
- *Stimulate natural action of intestines*
- *Protect intestinal canal from putrefactive or pathogenic bacteria*
- *Lower the cholesterol and triglyceride levels in the body*
- *Help prevent diabetes, ischemic heart disease, gallbladder disorders, varicose veins, diverticulitis, and appendicitis*

Suggested Use: 6–8 capsules two to three times daily 6 capsules daily will last: 33 days 7 capsules daily will last: 28 days 8 capsules daily will last: 25 days
Size Available: 200 capsules (450mg each)
Shelf Life: 7 years

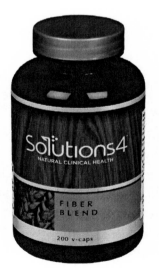

FIBER is an important part of the Solutions4 Detoxification Program.

Ingredients:
WHEAT BRAN POWDER — Insoluble fiber that scrubs the colon and adds bulk to stool. Does not absorb.
PSYLLIUM HUSK POWDER — Soluble fiber that absorbs toxins and helps scrub the colon. Psyllium provides 8 times more soluble fiber than oat bran.

DIGESTIVE ENZYME BLEND

The Solutions4 DIGESTIVE ENZYME BLEND provides a blend of natural digestive enzymes to supplement those provided by foods and the body itself. Taken with each meal, this formula is a preventive tool, assisting digestion, alleviating gastrointestinal discomfort and restoring energy to the body to improve overall health.

Helps the Body To:
- *Rest vital digestive organs*
- *Reduce probability of cancer, diabetes, heart disease, ulcers and other diet-related disorders*
- *Restore natural energy*
- *Increase immune system efficiency*
- *Reduce allergies and arthritis*
- *Promote weight control by heightening absorption of vitamins, minerals and other nutrients from food*
- *Help prevent turmoil caused by poor digestion: gas and bloating, diarrhea, constipation, heartburn, and insomnia*
- *Aid proper elimination*

Suggested Use: 1–2 capsules prior to each meal 1
capsule three times daily will last: 30 days
2 capsules three times daily will last: 15 days
Size Available: 90 capsules
Shelf Life: 4 years

Ingredients:
PROTEASE — Digests proteins (meat, beans, etc.). Implicated in standard cellular function and plays a role in the reproductive system. Involved in the processes of inflammation, infection, blood clotting, and blood purification. Promotes acid balance in the stomach to help prevent ulcers.

AMYLASE — Digests carbohydrates, starches and sugars (potatoes, fruits, vegetables, breads, pasta, etc). Rests the pancreas because some of the amylase needed to digest carbohydrates comes from the pancreas.

LIPASE — Digests fats and oils (nuts, avocados, olives, etc.). Rests the gall bladder. Promotes cardiovascular health. Assists weight control.

CELLULASE — Digests fiber (fruits, vegetables, grain, etc.). Maximizes absorption of anthocyanidins, tremendous antioxidants from blueberries, grapes, and other berries.

SUCRASE — Digests sucrose (refined sugar).

MALTASE — Digests complex and simple carbohydrates (malt and grain sugars).

LACTASE — Digests lactose (milk sugar).

PANCREATIN — Aids in digestion and rests the pancreas because it is one of the digestive ferments of the pancreatic juice.

OMEGA 3 FATTY ACID — Helps reduce the possibility of cardiovascular disease. Promotes upper and lower gastrointestinal motility while enhancing nutrient absorption.

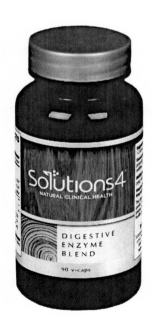

EVENING PRIMROSE OIL

Solutions4 EVENING RIMROSE OIL (EPO), comes from the seeds of the evening primrose plant. Once known chiefly for its beauty, few knew of its healing powers as an herb.

This Omega 6 fatty acid is a rich source of gamma linolenic acid (GLA), an essential fatty acid (EFA) that the body converts to a hormone-like substance called prostaglandin E1 (PGE1). Prostaglandins positively affect every organ of the body, and are especially beneficial to the heart, skin, and immune system. A shortage of prostaglandins results in impaired health. With an increase of GLA in the diet, the body is better able to function and properly fight disease.

Evening Primrose Oil has been shown to:

- Lower weight without dieting
- Lower blood cholesterol
- Lower blood pressure
- Heal or improve eczema
- Lesson rheumatoid arthritis
- Normalize saliva and tear production
- Relieve premenstrual pain
- Slow progression of multiple sclerosis
- Improve acne when taken with zinc
- Improve function of hyperactive children
- Strengthen fingernails
- Alleviate hangovers

Suggested Use: Take 3–6 softgels daily 3
softgels daily will last: 66 days 6
softgels daily will last: 33 days
Amount varies according to the nutritional program you are on.
Speak to your nutritional counselor.
Size Available: 200 softgels (500mg each)
Shelf Life: 3 years

Ingredients:

EVENING PRIMROSE OIL — A natural oil known to improve overall health and alleviate discomforts from many health conditions, including PMS, eczema, breast pain and rheumatoid arthritis.

LINOLEIC ACID — Enhances muscle growth, lowers cholesterol and triglycerides, reduces food-induced allergic reactions and enhances immune system.

GAMMA LINOLENIC ACID (GLA) — May help: heart disease, lupus, osteoarthritis, rheumatoid arthritis, diabetes, eczema, fingernail problems, endometriosis, menstrual cramps, premenstrual syndrome, and sunburn.

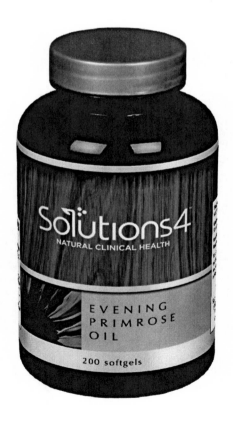

FLAX SEED OIL

The seeds and oil of the flax plant contain substances which promote good health. Flax seed oil is rich in alphalinolenic acid (ALA), which belongs to a group of substances called omega-3 fatty acids. Omega-3 is beneficial to the heart, helping to protect against heart disease and control high blood pressure.

Flax seed oil contains lignans, which may have antioxidant actions and protect against breast, colon, prostate, and skin cancer. Studies have shown flaxseed to slow down the division of tumor cells.

Omega-3s have been shown to counter the inflammatory response, which is helpful to those with inflammatory conditions such as lupus and gout.

Suggested Use:
Take 2–6 softgels daily. For best absorption, take with food. 2 softgels daily will last: 60 days 4 softgels daily will last: 30 days 6 softgels daily will last: 20 days
Size Available: 120 softgels (1000mg each)
Shelf Life: 3 years

Ingredients:
- ORGANIC FLAX SEED OIL
- Which typically contains:
- ALPHA-LINOLENIC ACID (omega 3) — 585 mg
- LINOLEIC ACID (omega 3) — 150 mg
- OLEIC ACID (omega 9) — 175 mg
- OTHER FATTY ACIDS/ PHYTONUTRIENTS — 90 mg

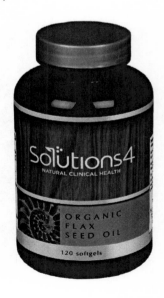

HERBAL STRESS RELIEF

Offers natural stress relief while helping the body maintain and/or restore maximum performance balance.

Solutions4 HERBAL STRESS RELIEF is an enhanced Valerian Root Formula which acts as a natural and relaxing stress-reliever. Valerian is a perennial plant found in New England and Europe. The root has been blended with Hops Flowers, Chamomile Flowers, and Passion Flowers in a synergistic formula. These ingredients have traditionally been used for relaxation.

Suggested Use: 2 capsules daily, one capsule morning and one capsule evening (more may be taken if desired. Do not exceed 12 capsules in one 24-hour period)

2 capsules daily will last: 45 days

Size Available: 90 capsules

Shelf Life: 7 years

Ingredients:

PASSION FLOWER — Sedative, calms the nervous system and promotes sleep.

VALERIAN ROOT — Very potent tranquilizer, antispasmodic, and mild anodyne.

CHAMOMILE FLOWER — Sedative, good for excitement and nervous stomach.

HOPS FLOWERS — Sedative, restoring tonic for the nervous system.

CATNIP — Antispasmodic, digestive stimulant, promotes cooling.

LAVENDER FLOWER — Sedative and analgesic; antispasmodic.

MYRRH GUM — Immune stimulant, circulatory stimulant.

SPEARMINT LEAVES — Antispasmodic, digestive tonic, promotes bile flow. Relaxes peripheral blood vessels.

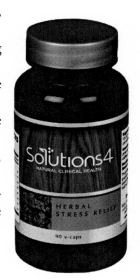

HORMONE BALANCE

Solutions4 HORMONE BALANCE is a safe and natural way to stabilize the hormones of the body for both women and men. This formula is an alternative to synthetic hormones, as it allows the body to produce and regulate its own hormonal balance.

Features and Benefits of HORMONE BALANCE:
For Women:
    Helps assist with a healthy menstrual cycle
    Helps with symptoms of PMS, including:
    Cramping1.
    Menopause2.
    Vaginal dryness3.
For Men:
    Increases effect of testicular hormones
    Suggested Use: 2–3 capsules twice daily 2
    capsules twice daily will last: 45 days3
    capsules twice daily will last: 30 days
    Size Available: 180 capsules
    Shelf Life: 7 years

Ingredients:
    BLESSED THISTLE — Used for treating painful menstruation .

    DAMIANA — Used to improve sexual potency , aphrodisiac , relieves headaches.

    DONG QUAI EXTRACT — Anti-spasmodic. Treatment of hormone symptoms such as hot flashes, menopause, vaginal dryness, PMS. Increases the effect of ovarian / testicular hormones.

    KAVA KAVA — Potent analgesic — used for vaginitis and urinary tract. Sedative, muscular relaxant for relief of insomnia, stress, anxiety.

    SERENOA SERRULATA — Prostate, irritable bladder relief.

    WILD YAM EXTRACT — Progesterone precursor, treats nausea in pregnancy, active agent in hormone precursors.

MOTHERWORT — Used to treat suppressed menstruation and other female disorders , used to treat nervous conditions , thyroid, hypertension.

LICORICE ROOT — High in calcium , tissue nourishing tonic, aids hypoglycemia, nausea, promotes adrenal gland function, helps with menopausal ailments. Estrogen effects.

BLACK COHOSH — Anti-spasmodic , diuretic , influences the nervous system. Used in menstrual and uterine affections.

RED RASPBERRY LEAF — Antispasmodic , for disorders of gastrointestinal tract, morning sickness, hot flashes, cramps, decreases heavy menstrual flow.

PASSION FLOWER — For nervous agitation, mild insomnia, depression.

CRAMP BARK — Antispasmodic, diuretic tonic, sedative, prevents miscarriage, dysmenorrhea, ovarian irritation, cramps.

PARSLEY — Flushing, helpful for urinary tract, bladder inflammation.

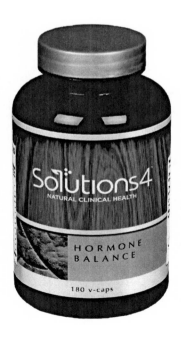

INTESTINAL CLEANSER

Solutions4 INTESTINAL CLEANSER is part of a complete Detoxification program. This is a program which temporarily replaces a normal diet of solid food, utilizing liquid food and cleansing supplements to detoxify the body systems.

INTESTINAL CLEANSER is an herbal bowel tonic that helps break down hard encrustation of waste for removal from the colon during Detoxification , as well as on its own for effective and healthy elimination.

- *Safe tonic-laxative*
- *Increases circulation to bowels*
- *Lubricates the intestinal tract*
- *Aids in healing bowels*
- *Relieves gas and pains in the bowels*
- *Will expel worms from intestines*
- *Powerful anti-inflammatory and anti-irritant for joints and the gastro-intestinal tract*
- *High in minerals including iron*
- *Improves function of the stomach and liver*

An important part of the Solutions4 DETOXIFICATION program

Suggested Use: 2–3 capsules twice daily
When utilized in a 30-day program, 120 capsules will be used
2 capsules twice daily will last: 22 days 3
capsules twice daily will last: 15 days

Dosage will be adjusted accordingly when taken as a part of the Detoxification Program. As a special dietary supplement, take 2-3 capsules twice daily with a large glass of water.

Size Available: 90 capsules
Shelf Life: 7 years

Ingredients:

CASCARA SAGRADA BARK — One of the safest tonic-laxative herbs known, and can be used on a daily basis without becoming habit forming. Stimulates secretions of the entire digestive system.

CLOVES — Increases circulation, improves digestion. Anti-spasmodic, relieving pain by reducing cramping in muscles. Affects nerves directly, reducing pain signals to the brain.

FENNEL SEED — Relieves gas and pains in the bowels. Has a cooling affect on the bowels. Lubricates the intestines and is very healing.

GINGER ROOT — Eliminates and counteracts the formation of mucus. Taken to relieve gas and severe pains in the bowels. Destroys parasites in the digestive system. Increases energy of the body. Stimulates circulation and breaks up obstructions.

YELLOW DOCK ROOT — An astringent blood purifier useful in treating diseases of the blood, and chronic skin ailments. Stimulates digestion, improving the function of the stomach and liver.

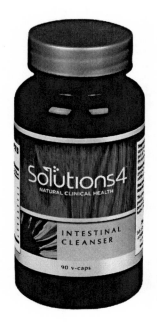

MARSHMALLOW ROOT — Powerful anti-inflammatory and an anti-irritant for joints and the gastro-intestinal tract. High in minerals, especially easily assimilable calcium. Used for chronic constipation. Protective and healing in intestinal irritations.

BUTTERNUT BARK — Will expel worms from intestines. Remedy for chronic constipation.

LICORICE ROOT — Helps eliminate built up toxins. Constipation is considered a serious problem because the retention of wastes in the body can lead to more serious diseases. Used to protect damaged or inflamed tissues.

JOINT & MUSCLE RELIEF

A natural treatment for arthritis, stiffness, swollen joints, and muscular aches and pains. Solutions4 JOINT & MUSCLE RELIEF assists in body healing through a combination of herbs that help rebuild and strengthen body tissue, increase joint lubrication, and reduce inflammation around the joints.

Natural treatment for:
- Arthritis
- Stiffness of the joints
- Swollen joints
- Muscular aches and pains

Assists Body Healing By:
- Cleansing accumulated toxins and wastes
- Strengthening all vital organs
- Helping glands to revitalize themselves
- Re-establishing chemical balance in the tissues
- Rebuilding and strengthening general health of the body

Suggested Use: 2–3 capsules three times daily
- 2 capsules three times daily will last: 33 days
- 3 capsules three times daily will last: 22 days
- Size Available: 200 capsules
- Shelf Life: 7 years

Ingredients:

ALFALFA — Used in the recovery of acute ailments and in rebuilding energy. A blood purifier, used to treat toxicity of blood, arthritis and cancer.

YUCCA — Helps flush excess water from the system. Assists in excretion of bile salt and cholesterol into the intestines. Helps in the reduction of swelling.

LICORICE ROOT — Treats adrenal insufficiency. Has a

stimulating action and helps counteract stress.

BURDOCK ROOT & SEED — A valuable purifier, used for the treatment of arthritis, rheumatism, sciatica and lumbago. Promotes kidney function, working through the kidneys to help clear the blood of harmful acids.

SARSPARILLA — Useful in the treatment of gout, rheumatism, colds, fever, ringworm, skin eruptions, as well as other ailments requiring a good blood purifier.

DEVILS CLAW ROOT — Anti-inflammatory in joints, hepatic tonic, diuretic, sedative, lymphatic stimulant.

PRICKLY ASH — Digestive stimulant, alterative especially for the joints, diaphoretic, peripheral circulatory stimulant.

ASCORBIC ACID (Vitamin C) — Assists in rebuilding the immune system.

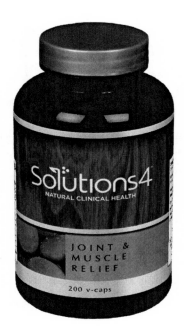

MULTIVITAMIN / MULTIMINERAL

Solutions4 MULTIVITAMIN / MULTIMINERAL is the perfect combination of essential vitamins and minerals that are necessary for health. This formula utilizes the process of chelation, which binds minerals with amino acids, making assimilation by the body much more efficient than comparable supplements.

The Importance of Chelation:

MULTIVITAMIN / MULTIMINERAL is an important and effective formula because of its chelation. [Key'lation] This is the process by which mineral substances are changed into their digestible form. Common mineral supplements such as bone meal and dolomite are often not chelated and must first be acted upon in the digestive process to form chelates before they are of use to the body.

The natural chelating process is not performed efficiently in many people, and because of this, many of the mineral supplements they take are of little use.

It is important to understand that the body does not use everything it takes in, and that most of us do not digest our foods efficiently. Additionally, only two to ten percent of inorganic iron taken into the body is actually absorbed, and even with this small percentage, 50 percent is then eliminated.

Taking all these factors into account, you can recognize the importance of ingesting minerals that have been chelated. Amino acid-bound chelated mineral supplements provide three to ten times greater assimilation than those that are non-chelated.

Suggested Use:
- 1 capsule twice daily, one morning and night 1
- capsule twice daily will last: 45 days
- Sizes Available: 90 capsules
- Shelf Life: 2-3 years

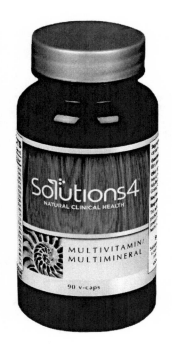

Ingredients:

Vitamins A, C, D, E, B1, B2, B3, B6, B12, Niacin, Calcium Pantothenate, Folic Acid, Biotin, Inositol, Choline, PABA, Lipotropic, Calcium Chelate, Potassium, Magnesium Chelate, Manganese Chelate, Zinc Chelate, Alfalfa, Kelp, Phosphorus, Pantothenic Acid, Iron Chelate, Chronium Chelate, Molybdenum, Iodine, Selenium

NUTRITIONAL SHAKE

This candida-friendly shake mixes instantly with water or milk, and can be used as a perfectly balanced meal replacement when you are on the go. The Solutions4 NUTRITIONAL SHAKE can also be a part of a healthy weight loss program by becoming a substitute for two out of three meals a day while providing essential nutrients to the body. Available in chocolate, vanilla, strawberry and orange cream.

Features and Benefits

- Easy mixing
- Great taste
- No artificial sweeteners
- Low glycemic ratio
- Contains digestive enzymes, probiotics, omega 3 fatty acids and trace minerals
- Lactose, soy and gluten free as well as candida friendly

Suggested Use: For meal replacement, use 2 level scoops mixed with 8 oz of water. For a healthy snack in-between meals, mix 1 level scoop with 4-6 oz. of water. You may substitute all or some of the water with rice milk or almond milk. For variety, try adding frozen berries, fresh fruit and/or ice.

- 1 scoop 1 time daily will last: 30 days
- 2scoops 1 time daily will last: 15 days
- Size Available: 22.75 oz (15 meals or 30 snacks)
- Shelf Life: 6 years

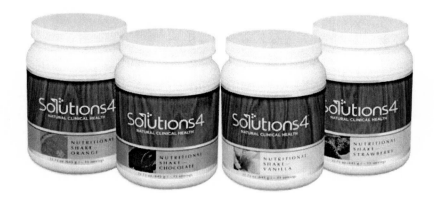

Ingredients:

VITAMIN A, C, E, K, B1, B2, B5, B6, B12, K, CALCIUM, FOLIC ACID, MAGNESIUM, CLA, ACIDOPHILUS & BIFIDUS, OMEGA 3 FATTY ACIDS, PROBIOTIC BLEND, BIOTIN, CHROMIUM, IRON, NIACINAMIDE, POTASSIUM, XYLITOL, DIGESTIVE ENZYME BLEND

PROBIOTIC BLEND

Solutions4 PROBIOTIC BLEND contains friendly microbes to control the population of hostile bacteria and yeast, especially after times of intense stress, infection, antibiotic therapy, or any event that may cause immune system depletion. Probiotics are also known to maintain or revive overall health. This specialized formula is enteric-coated which insures that the formula will be absorbed only where it is needed most — within the intestines.

The Solutions4 Formula:

This probiotic formulation helps to maintain healthy intestinal activity. The function of the human digestive system is to convert the food we eat into useful body fuel. A necessary and healthful contributor to a properly working digestive system is an abundant supply of the "friendly" bacteria. Solutions4 PROBIOTIC BLEND contains 4 friendly bacteria for this purpose.

This is an effective alternative to all candida albicans prescription drugs, and it causes no side effects. The Solutions4 formula is patient-tested and proven effective in chiropractic and wellness clinics.

PROBIOTIC BLEND contains 20 billion units per serving (10 billion units per capsule).

Features and Benefits
- Helps to maintain healthy intestinal activity
- Prevents the overgrowth of harmful micro-organisms
- Helps prevent bad breath, gas and bloating
- Improves the overall health of the skin by combating harmful bacteria

Suggested Use:
- 1–2 capsules four times daily as needed
- 1 capsule four times daily will last: 22 days
- 2 capsules four times daily will last: 11 days
- Size Available: 90 capsules
- Shelf Life: 4 years

Ingredients:

VITAMIN A (BETA-CAROTENE) — Promotes growth, strong bones, and healthy skin, hair, teeth, eyes, and gums.

VITAMIN C (ASCORBIC ACID) — Aids in preventing many types of viral and bacterial infections and generally strengthens the immune system.

BIOTIN — A B-vitamin that is needed for the formation of fatty acids and glucose, which are essential for the production of energy. It also helps with the metabolism of carbohydrates, fats and proteins.

ZINC CITRATE — Fights infection and stimulates the immune system.

LACTOBACILLUS ACIDOPHILUS — Friendly bacteria normally found in the intestinal tract, which are necessary and healthful contributors to a properly working digestive system.

BARBERRY ROOT — Helps to build the immune system and prevent yeast overgrowth.

LICORICE — Works by promoting the overall health of the gastrointestinal system.

PAU D'ARCO — An effective anti-fungal herb.

GARLIC — Creates an atmosphere that prohibits bacteria and fungus. (Candida is a form of fungus.)

GOLDENSEAL ROOT — Helps to destroy bacteria and viruses, as well as helps to relieve inflammation and congestion.

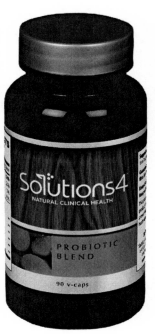

SALMON OIL

Wild salmon oil does not suffer from the faults that plague traditional fish oils. A salmon's cold-water habitat and relatively short lifespan dramatically reduce the exposure to common environmental toxins, resulting in a higher quality, higher purity oil.

A salmon's high dietary intake of protective carotenoids such as astaxanthin make their oil more resistant to spoilage and rancidity than other fish oils. Salmon are a renewable, self sustaining resource. Other fish oils, which are commonly a blend of several species of fish, have a much less consistent level and blend of healthy omega acids, especially epa and dha. Each serving of salmon oil containg 180 mg of epa and 220 mg of dha, two of the most beneficial constituents of omega 3 fatty acid.

Salmon Oil has been shown to:

- *Boost levels of HDL (good cholesterol) and lower the levels of triglycerides*
- *Aid in Healthy Aging*
- *Lower weight without dieting*
- *Increase Bone and Joint Health*
- *Assist in Cognitive Function*
- *Increase the health of the eyes, nails and skin*
- *Promotes healthy pregnancies and developing children*
- *Improve mental health*
- *Improve the health of the eyes, nails and skin*

Suggested Use:

Take 2 softgels 1/2 hour after breakfast and 2 softgels 1/2 hour after an evening meal.

- 4 capsules daily will last: 30 days
- Size Available: 120 capsules
- Shelf Life: 7 years

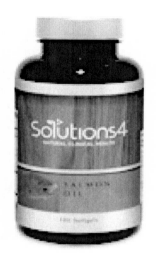

Ingredients:

SALMON OIL – Oil derived from Salmon containing high levels of Omega 3 fatty acids which contribute to the improvement of overall health.

During the processing of Solutions4's Salmon Oil, all mercury content was removed.

THYROID/ADRENAL

This unique formula was developed to benefit anyone suspecting a thyroid condition, as well as those seeking a daily supplement to ensure nutritional support of the thyroid and adrenals.

Solutions4 THYROID Adrenal Support stimulates healthy glandular function and contains a synergistic blend of herbs including kelp and bladderwrack, two potent sources of iodine which support your body's natural ability to produce thyroid hormones.

THYROID helps to restore the body's optimal thyroid hormone level, and alleviate the symptoms of thyroid disorders, such as: weight gain, low energy, fatigue and depression.

Suggested Use:

- 2 capsules, 2-3 times daily
- 4 capsules daily will last: 15 days
- 6 capsules daily will last: 10 days
- Size Available: 60 capsules
- Shelf Life: 7 years

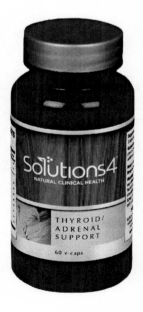

Ingredients:

KELP - A great source of natural iodine, potassium, magnesium, calcium, iron, B-complex vitamins, and 70 other micronutrients. Stimulates healthy thyroid function and improved metabolism.

COLEUS FORSKOHLII -Beneficial in fat loss due to its ability to break down adipose tissue, and discourage the formation of new fatty tissues. Directly stimulates the increased production of thyroid hormones.

BACOPA – A potent ayurvedic herb with antioxidant properties, bacopa helps to relieve stress and boost mental function.

HOPS FLOWER – An herbal stress reliever and hormonal support agent.

SAGE –Helps to control stress, improve digestion, and stimulate pancreatic function.

ASHWAGANDHA ROOT – An adaptogenic herb which helps to control stress and anxiety, and acts as a powerful anti-inflammatory, anti-oxidant, and immune system boost.

ROSEMARY– Helps to reduce stress, anti-oxidant.

BLADDERWRACK – A great source of natural iodine, calcium, magnesium, potassium, and B-complex vitamins. Stimulates healthy thyroid function.

GINSENG – An adaptogenic herb that aids in the control of high blood sugar. Boosts sports performance and recovery.

SCHIZANDRA ROOT – An adaptogenic, anti-oxidant herb. Helps with stress relief and boosts sports performance and recovery.

VITAMIN D

Studies have shown that adequate amounts of vitamin D in the body can decrease the risk of diseases, such as cancer, osteoporosis, depression, Alzheimer's and many others. Solutions4 VITAMIN D, in an easily-absorbed liquid gel form, and offers many health benefits, including:

- *Bone strengthening*
- *Lower risk of disease and infection*
- *Immune boosting*
- *Decrease cognitive decline with aging*

Suggested Use: 1–2 softgels, one time daily
  1 softgel daily will last: 150 days
  2 softgels daily will last: 75 days
  Size Available: 150 softgels (1000 IU each)
  Shelf Life: 7 years

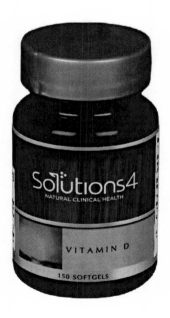

Ingredients:
VITAMIN D3 (Cholecalciferol) — The most potent form of supplemental vitamin D. 1000 IU per day provides enough vitamin D to rectify most deficiencies and supply the body with optimal levels of this beneficial immune-boosting nutrient.

BODY WRAP CREAM (Regular and Sensitive formulas)

Solutions4's BODY WRAP CREAM, promotes a healthy and permanent inch loss of 4-14 inches per treatment while maintaining proper hydration. Since this is not a water loss wrap, the inches lost will remain lost with a healthy diet and exercise. When utilized with a Body Wrap, excess cream will be absorbed by the skin eliminating the need of a wet room. This cream is very effective for those suffering from poor circulation and fluid retention.

BODY WRAP CREAM Helps to:
- Remove cellulite by targeting and removing the toxins trapped in the connective tissue
- Soothe, heal and stimulate new tissue growth
- Increase skin elasticity and improve skin's firmness
- Suggested Use: Client may have 1 body wrap every 4-7 days by a technician that has been certified in Solutions4's Body Contour and Inch Loss Programs.

Size Available: 2 oz = 1 body wrap
Quart = 16 body wraps
Gallon = 64 body wraps
Available in regular and sensitive formulas.
Proffesional Use Only
Shelf Life: 6 months - 1 year

Ingredients:
NIACIN/ NIACINAMINDE — Niacin/Niacinamide: Increases circulation by dilating blood vessels while encouraging lymphatic flow.

SOY OIL — Helps to stimulate the synthesis of collagen, elastin, and structural glyco-proteins. Also helps to soothe the skin while providing essential nutrients such as vitamins A, E and K, phosphates and lecithin.

Wrap should never be performed on one who is pregnant, nursing or if one has not been in remission from cancer for 5 years or more. Also those on blood thinning medications such as Coumadin and those who suffer from seizures should not utilize body contouring products.

ANTI-CELLULITE LOTION

Solutions4 ANTI-CELLULITE lotion has the ability to maximize and preserve the contouring, tightening and inch loss achieved through the Solutions4 Body Contour

Wrap. Essential nutrients increase circulation, helping to condition and tone the skin. Active ingredients are retained in concentrated levels to assist in the cleansing and cellulite removal process, leaving the skin with a delicate cinnamon scent.

Helps to:
- Increase circulation
- Soften and condition the skin
- Tighten and tone
- Aid in the removal of cellulite

Suggested Use: Anti-Cellulite Lotion should be applied immediately after showering or bathing, on all days in between body wraps or as an everyday lotion. (Before initial use it is advised that a patch test be performed at least 8 hours prior to application.) Apply to dry skin in a circular motion, treating the problem areas of the hips, buttocks, thighs, upper arms, etc. Avoid breasts and bikini areas.

Please Note: Due to increased circulation the skin may become pink immediately following application, normal coloring will return shortly following use.

Size Available: 8 ounce & Quart
Shelf Life: 1 year

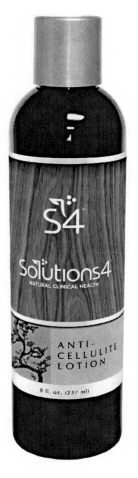

Ingredients:

ALOE VERA: A botanical extract which helps to calm, heal and soothe the skin. It is also considered
natures anti-biotic, working as an antibacterial, anti-inflammatory, and as an anti-fungal.

VITAMIN A: Improves skin texture and firmness, helps to fade and prevent discolorations. Converts
to retinoic acid which renews skin by promoting cell turnover and provides anti-aging benefits.

CUCUMBER EXTRACT: Helps to tighten and firm the skin while binding moisture, healing and
combating inflammation.

BODY EXFOLIATOR

Solutions4's Body Exfoliator is a superior enzymatic and manual exfoliator that utilizes papaya enzymes which dissolve dead skin and round pumice crystals that exfoliate. This formula is unique and unlike sea salt will not cut or damage the skin's surface. This gentle exfoliant softens the skin and delays the appearance of fine lines and wrinkles.

Helps to:

Remove dead cells
Dilate capillaries which enables nutrients to get to the cells
Stimulate the metabolism of the skin
Activate the M'lis body CONTOUR cream

Suggested Use:

Apply to the body three times weekly with or without water. May be applied to dry skin before showering, rubbing in circular motion from feet to shoulders, or use on wet skin in the shower for less intensity. Not for use on the face.

Sizes Available: 8 ounce & Quart
Shelf Life: 1 year

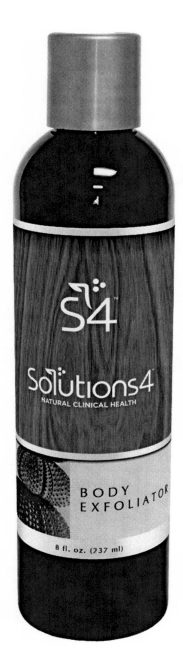

Ingredients:

ALOE VERA - A botanical extract which helps to calm, heal and soothe the skin. It is also considered natures anti-biotic, working as an anti-bacterial, anti-inflammatory, and as an anti-fungal.

ROUNDED PUMICE (volcanic origin) - An abrasive exfoliant used to remove dead skin cells.

BETA GLUCAN - Stimulates formation of collagen.

PAPAIN - Live papaya enzymes act as a gentle exfoliant which help to dissolve dead skin cells and encourage deeper penetration for additional products.

GERANIUM EXTRACT - Works as an astringent while aiding in cell regeneration.

CYPRESS SAGE EXTRACT - Has antiseptic and astringent properties helping to soothe the skin.

Also available for professional use- Use prior to Body Wrap. This synergistic formula activates the M'lis CONTOUR CREAM and Solutions4's Maintain Lotion for deeper penetration to achieve maximum inch loss.

EXERCISE GEL

Solutions4 EXERCISE GEL applied before exercise, improves pre-exercise stretching and encourages mobility and circulation throughout a workout. The ingredients in Solutions4 EXERCISE GEL are scientifically formulated to cause the blood to flow more quickly and evenly into the connective tissues. Circulation helps the body's waste disposal system to more efficiently expel toxic waste and fluid, sculpting and toning vulnerable cellulite areas. EXERCISE GEL is also used for sore muscles, fibromyalgia, arthritis, and aching joints, to encourage a more productive and comfortable exercise session. Natural herbal extracts are safe for all skin types and can be used with any kind of exercise, including meditation and yoga.

Helps to:

- Keep muscles warm and moveable
- Increase circulation
- Expel toxic waste and fluid

Suggested Use: Apply EXERCISE GEL to the problem areas of the body, any sore muscles or joints, or anywhere that the client wishes to reduce tissue toxins. It can be used up to three times daily with or without exercise for improved circulation and mobility.

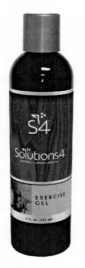

Size Available: 8 ounce & Quart
Shelf Life: 1 year

Ingredients:
ALOE VERA - A botanical extract which helps to calm, heal and soothe the skin. It is also considered natures anti-biotic, working as an antibacterial, anti-inflammatory, and as an anti-fungal.
BLADDERWRACK EXTRACT - Works on the glandular system.
ALLANTOIN - A natural botanical extract which heals and sooths the skin while working to calm irritation and stimulate new tissue growth.
NIACIN - Increases circulation by dilating blood vessels while increasing lymphatic flow which assists in removing toxins from connective tissue.

CHAPTER
ELEVEN

Additional Resources

REJUVENATION PROGRAM

with Self-Mastery Technology™
Patrick K. Porter, Ph.D. & Todd Singleton, D.C.

The Club Reduce doctors spent over 20 years researching and testing methods that promote healing and weight reduction. The self-mastery program you are about to embark upon is all about getting you results. We partnered with mind-based wellness expert Patrick K. Porter, Ph.D. because our goal at Club Reduce is to help the body heal itself naturally. We know this can only happen when both your body and mind are engaged in the

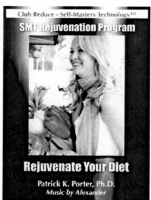

healing process. This program is the "missing link" to weight loss because it retrains your brain while you are retraining your body. When your body and mind are truly healthy, you will arrive at your proper weight. With the help of Dr. Porter's super-learning technology, we will educate you on how to live a new and improved lifestyle from the inside out. Our goal is to have you thinking, eating and responding to life as a naturally thin, healthy-minded person—now that's true self-mastery!

RVP01 – Rejuvenate Your Diet

When not detoxifying or juicing, your diet should consist mostly of green leafy vegetables. During this session, you will be guided to design a lifestyle of health and vitality in which you easily incorporate more greens into your diet. You will use the power of your imagination to create an internal timeline in which you plan meals around salads. As you learn to think like a thin person, your daily intake of fruits and vegetables will increase naturally. As your thinking changes and as your weight reduces, you will eliminate the thinking that put the weight on in the first place.

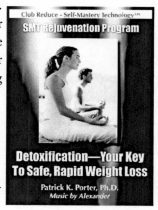

RVP02 – Detoxification—Your Key To Safe, Rapid Weight Loss

Detoxification is one of the most important factors in the promotion of good health and disease prevention. During this session, you will build the motivation to stick to your cleanse. As your body cleanses itself of toxins, mucus and other waste materials in the intestinal tract and major vital organs, improving the way they function, your positive attitude about your body and your life will improve as well, restoring vital energy to the organs and the entire body. The key here is to rid your body of toxins while cleansing your mind of any stinkin' thinkin'.

RVP03 – Prepare Yourself For A Healing Breakthrough

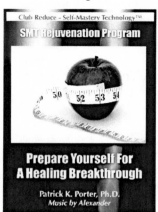

During detoxification and the days that follow, many people experience some of the signs of a healing crisis, which may include: headaches, skin breakouts, bowl sluggishness, diarrhea, fatigue, sweating, frequent urination, congestion, nasal discharge, or body aches. During this SMT session, you will create the mental toughness to transform the healing crisis into a health breakthrough. You will learn to relax and be patient with your body as it goes through cleansing and detoxification. You will become motivated to drink water to assist your body in its natural healing process and to use your SMT sessions to engage the amazing power of your mind.

RVP04 – The Supplement Solution

Appetite happens in the mind and hunger happens in the body. Once your body gets the nutrition it needs, and your mind gets the positive stimulation it needs, you'll find it easy to eliminate emotional eating.

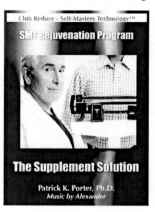

Once you're eating to satisfy physical hunger, and not the appetite, sticking to the rejuvenation program will be a breeze. The doctors at Club Reduce searched the globe for the highest quality products and chose only those that have a direct benefit to your health. This visualization will help you get and stay motivated about using supplements for vibrant good health. While listening, you will come to understand that this will not only help you lose the weight you want, but also improve every other aspect of your life.

CANDIDA HEALING BREAKTHROUGH
with Self-Mastery Technology™ (SMT)
Patrick K. Porter, Ph.D. & Todd Singleton, D.C.

At Club Reduce, our goal is to help your body heal itself naturally. We know this can only be accomplished when both your body and mind are engaged in the healing process. For this reason, we provide you with our exclusive Club Reduce SMT series: Candida Healing Breakthrough. Throughout this program, based on the principles of Dr. Todd Singleton's Club Reduce program, Dr. Patrick Porter will guide you on mental journeys that not only fully relax your body and mind, but also positively transform the internal landscape of your thoughts and beliefs relating to food, health, and healing. Throughout this series you will...

- *Take your commitment to new heights*
- *Reverse the negative side effects of stress*
- *Tame the tension tiger*
- *Eliminate emotional and stress eating habits*
- *Overcome negative lifestyle habits*
- *Restore normal, rejuvenating sleep patterns*
- *Supercharge your motivation*
- *Lock in healthy eating habits for life*

Each session will guide you on a mental vacation while building internal resources so you look forward to and enjoy your healthy daily activities. You'll feel a brand new level of confidence emerging until you know, without a doubt, that you will achieve your proper weight and vibrant good health. Soon the lifestyle habit of eating to live instead of living to eat will be as easy as taking a breath in open air.

The doctors at Club Reduce spent over 20 years researching and testing their methods with thousands of members. When you engage the power of your mind and imagination to model other successful members, you have every reason to expect the same excellent results!

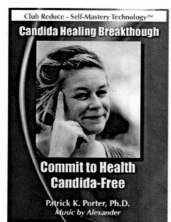

CHB01
Commit to Health Candida-Free

This opening session is all about reinforcing the exciting new information you're learning in your Club Reduce educational program. This session will not only help you lose the weight you want, but also improve every other aspect of your life. After relaxing with this session, your new and improved lifestyle will seem simple, easy and natural.

CHB02 – Stay On Track with Your "Get Fit" Food List

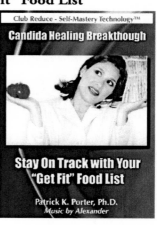

If all you need is a little motivation, this session is for you. It will provide you the incentive to succeed day by day, giving you the optimistic attitude for steadily slimming down and getting healthier. Staying free from candida is about being vigilant about your body's health. During this session, you will learn mental toughness that allows you to say yes when appropriate and empowers you to say no when appropriate.

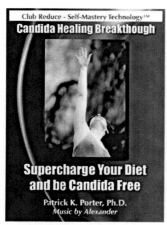

CHB03
Supercharge Your Diet and be Candida Free

Reducing is easy when you have a genuine desire for the natural ingredients that heal your body. This session will help you build a desire for the foods recommended in the breakthrough program while eliminating your desire for junk food. You deserve the highest quality of life possible—all you have to do is access the power in your own mind.

During this discovery, you will follow the preventive health approach, using nutrition and positive thinking to fight off disease and eliminate excess body weight, thus supercharging your results!

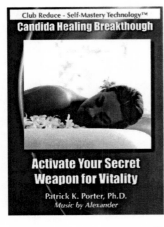

CHB04
Activate Your Secret Weapon for Vitality

Your future is yours for the making! In this session, you will create a timeline for success in which you beautify and better your body with the researched methods in the Candida Breakthrough Program. This process will assist you in using your body's ability to heal naturally. Rather than trying to force the body by using harmful chemicals, surgery, or addictive drugs, you will use nature as your secret weapon for achieving true health and vitality. You will sleep better, knowing that you are a lifetime partner with your body in maintaining a healthy and vitality-driven lifestyle.

CHB05 – From Healing Crisis to Total Rejuvenation

Candida Albicans is an over-infestation of yeast in the body. It can invade the brain and every tissue. During this session, Dr. Porter will help you focus on the long-term benefits you will enjoy by completing your health and rejuvenation plan. Candida grows and lives on what you eat, and makes your body crave the foods that feed candida. Now you will engage the power of your mind and positive thinking to rid your body and mind of any desire for candida-causing foods. Candida is difficult to get rid of and can cause you to experience a healing crisis, but this session will help you transform that crisis into anticipation and excitement for the total health rejuvenation you are about to enjoy.

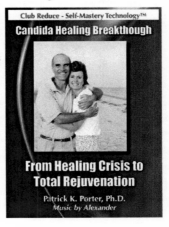

CHB06 – Eliminate the Foods that Destroy Friendly Bacteria

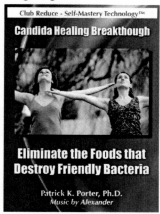

Sugar, gluten and meat encourage harmful bacterial growth in the intestines. During this session, you will learn the mental skills that make it easy to avoid these foods. Poor nutrition combined with a sluggish or impaired immune system weakens the body's ability to fight off yeast. But now, by achieving the relaxation response, you will empower your immune system to function as it was intended. Stress and environmental pollutants can also play a role in reducing the body's control over candida. You will rehearse coping skills to keep your body in balance, making it easy to say no to alcohol, caffeine and stress so friendly bacteria can thrive in your body.

CHB07 – Eradicate the Effects of Candida

Too much yeast can cripple the immune system, causing chronic viral and bacterial infection or allergies. Yeast can damage the intestinal wall, allowing food particles and toxins to enter the blood stream. The body then produces antibodies to fight these foreign substances and typical "allergic" reactions may occur, such as eczema and hay fever, along with headache, dizziness, heart palpitations, anxiety, fatigue, and muscle aches. This session will give you laser-like focus on eradicating the yeast, ridding yourself of these unwanted symptoms, and taking charge of your own health and quality of life. Step by step, you will reinforce the positive benefits of the candida breakthrough, allowing you to awaken from the session stress-free and with an unwavering determination to rid your body of candida for good.

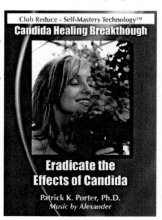

CHB08 –Stress-Free, Candida-Free

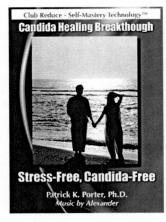

Stress can release powerful hormones that cause candida growth in the body. While listening to this session, you will reach a profound level of relaxation where you develop automatic responses for handling or eliminating anxiety, irritability, moodiness, restlessness, panic attacks, sudden anger, sleep disturbances, poor short-term memory, inability to concentrate, fuzzy thinking and confusion. Dr. Porter will also help you beat the fatigue that often accompanies impaired metabolism and poor enzyme production. The strategies you develop while relaxing with this session will help you safely eliminate unwanted weight for life.

CHB09 – Get Friendly with Friendly Bacteria

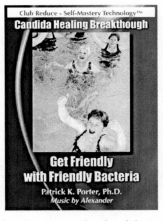

Friendly bacteria strains can suppress harmful bacteria. Through mental rehearsal, you will put behind you the bad habits that caused an unhealthy balance of bacteria in the first place. You will then use your newfound knowledge from the Candida Breakthrough Program to lock in the positive, empowering choices for a healthy balance of bacteria in your body. You will then build an automatic mechanism for desiring and choosing the natural foods that help friendly bacteria flourish. Keeping your body candida-free is easy when you build an internal mechanism for effortlessly choosing the health-building ingredients your body needs to reach complete wellness.

CHB10 –Enjoy Water – Nature's Elixir for Health

Water is critical to the treatment of any health condition, including candida. Every organ of the body requires water. During this session, you will build your desire for water and supercharge

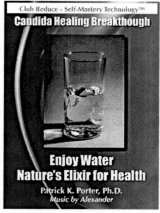

Enjoy Water
Nature's Elixir for Health

your motivation to drink all that your body needs for flushing toxins and healing every cell. Through the power of thought, you will build the habit of drinking water while regaining your taste for nature's health elixir. There are no substitutes for water, and soon you'll be that person who will not settle for less than the best for your body. Visualizing drinking enough water each day and then doing it will=have you feeling more energetic and positive than you've dreamed possible.

CHB11 – Unlock Your Body's Innate Healer

During this SMT session, Dr. Porter will help you tap into your inner healer. By following Club Reduce's core values of beautify and better the body through researched methods, this visualization will help you relax and let that power greater than yourself do the work. When you get out of the way and allow the Club Reduce program to do what it does naturally, your body's own ability to achieve optimum health will transform your experience—and isn't that better than harmful chemicals, surgery, or addictive drugs?

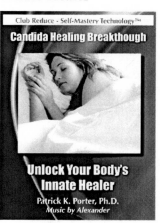

CHB12 – Put Your Candida-Free Lifestyle on Auto-Pilot

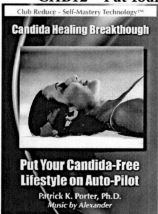

Dr. Porter will guide you through a timeline of change so that what you learned over the last 12 weeks will be locked into your mind and show up as new behaviors, a new attitude and positive core beliefs that will keep you candida free for life. You will experience the new energy and joy of taking back control. With this breakthrough lesson in life mastery, you will gain conscious tools to keep you on track with your health as naturally as you are breathing.

Dr. Patrick Porter's
Stress-Free Lifestyle Series

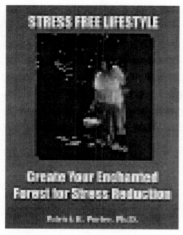

Stress is the most pervasive malady of our time. The effects on our health, productivity and quality of life are more devastating than most people care to admit. Luckily, you've just found the solution! SMT can help you see yourself as the healthy, happy, optimistic person you'd prefer to be. With this new image, your fears and frustrations fade away, your anxiety vanishes, and you no longer let small things stress you.

Create Your Enchanted Forest for Stress Reduction

Follow along as Dr. Patrick Porter guides you through your personal enchanted forest—a quiet, serene place where you have nothing to do but relax. Your other-than-conscious mind will massage away all tension, allowing you to release all negative thoughts and feelings. You'll return from your magical forest filled with positive feelings, able to enjoy and express your true inner peace.

Create Your Mountaintop Retreat for Stress Reduction

Say goodbye to all stress and confusion as you take a trip to this breathtaking mountaintop retreat. When you listen to this restful process, using your mind to relax your body will become as comfortable and automatic as breathing. The stress, strain and confusion of everyday life will melt away as you awake refreshed, revitalized and renewed!

A Complete List of
Stress-Free Titles
and full descriptions
can be found at
www.Self-MasteryTechnology.com

Dr. Patrick Porter's
Vibrant Health Series

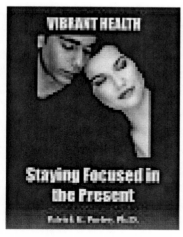

Of all the cells in your body, more than 50,000 will die and be replaced with new cells, all in the time it took you to read this sentence! Your body is the vehicle you have been given for the journey of your life. Dr. Patrick Porter will show you how, by using creative visualization and relaxation (SMT), you can recharge and energize your body, mind, and spirit. This series is for people who are looking for more than good health; it's for those who will settle for nothing less than vibrant health!

Staying Focused in the Present

Your emotions can either help your body stay healthy, or they can be the cause of disease. Negative feelings such as regret, worry, or anxiety about an upcoming event not only wastes your precious life, but also adds stress to the body, which makes you more susceptible to disease. In this SMT process, Dr. Porter will help you stay present and focused on the beauty of each moment and the gift each minute offers you.

Visualize a Heart-Healthy Lifestyle

Heart disease is not a male issue alone; it is the top killer of American women. To protect your heart, you need a plan that includes movement, a healthy diet, and a positive mental attitude. You use an average of forty-three muscles to frown and only seventeen muscles to smile. During this SMT session, Dr. Porter will show you how to celebrate the energy, passion, and power that are your birthright.

Check Out The Complete
Vibrant Health Series
www.Self-MasteryTechnology.com

Dr. Patrick Porter's
Life-Mastery Series

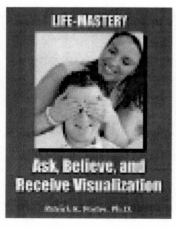

Throughout your life, from parents, teachers, and society, you were taught what to think. With the breakthrough processes of creative visualization and relaxation, you are going to discover how to think. With this knowledge you will literally become a software engineer for your own mind. On the Life-Mastery journey, you will explore the processes that best suit your needs for creating limitless personal improvement and success in your life.

Ask, Believe & Receive
Visualization

The universe operates on specific laws. These invisible laws are always manifesting your physical reality. The universe never tries anything; it only does. This visualization calls upon the Law of Attraction, and helps you to become a conscious creator. You will discover how you designed, at the core of your being, to be an active participant in the enfoldment of your relationships, wealth and happiness.

The Secret Power of Self-talk

On average, you give yourself over 5,000 messages a day. With this process you will discover how to weed your mental garden of negative thoughts and to sow new, more positive thoughts. You will use the same four-step process that has helped thousands of people neutralize fear, anxiety and worry. Using SMT, you discover the secret power of self-talk to easily create the habits, patterns, and beliefs that can put your success on autopilot.

Check Out The Complete
Life-Mastery Series
at www.Self-MasteryTechnology.com

Dr. Patrick Porter's
Wealth Consciousness Series

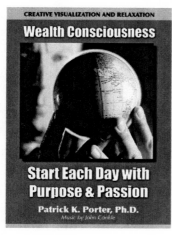

*Inspired by the principles
of Napoleon Hill's
Think and Grow Rich*

Start Each Day
with Purpose and Passion

Napoleon Hill understood that people don't plan to fail; they fail to plan. Successful people know where they are going before they start and move forward on their own initiative. They have the power of intention, or what Napoleon Hill called "mind energy," on their side.

Commit to a Life Spent with Like-Minded People

Together with Dr. Patrick Porter, you will use the power of intention to draw to yourself mastermind alliances that will support your dream. You will visualize setting up and using these mastermind alliances to help you attract goal-oriented people and create your success environment.

Trust the Power of
Infinite Intelligence

Do you sometimes feel as though negative thoughts and fear of poverty have control over you? During this SMT session, Dr. Porter will guide you through the principle of applied faith. All conditions are the offspring of thought, and you find it natural to visualize and realize the thoughts and actions that bring wealth and riches into your life.

Check Out The Complete
Wealth Consciousness Series
at www.Self-MasteryTechnology.com

Dr. Patrick Porter's
Weight Control Series

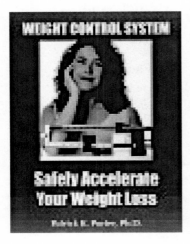

Now you can design the body you want and the life you love. That's right, you can have the trim, healthy body you've always dreamed of by simply changing the way you see yourself and your life. Once you have a new image of yourself, everything else changes—junk food and fast food lose their appeal, healthy foods become desirable, and you eat only when you're hungry. With Dr. Porter's System you will overcome common weight loss mistakes, learn to eat and think like a naturally thin person, conquer cravings, and increase your self-confidence. Each week you will take another step toward a lifetime of healthy living; losing weight is the natural byproduct of these changes. While the average diet lasts just 72 hours and focuses on depriving you of the foods you love, Dr. Patrick Porter supercharges your weight loss motivation with these powerful creative visualization and relaxation processes! You will eliminate the problem where it started—your own mind. There is simply no easier way to lose weight than SMT!

Safely Speeding Up Weight Loss

In this powerful process, you'll learn to safely speed up weight loss by thinking, acting and responding like a naturally thin person. Your sense of worth will improve when you discover and use inner resources you never even knew you had. Sit back, relax, and discover how easy it is to turn your body into a fat-burning machine—and keep the weight off forever!

Check Out The Complete
Weight Control Series
at **www.Self-MasteryTechnology.com**

Dr. Patrick Porter's
Accelerated Learning Series

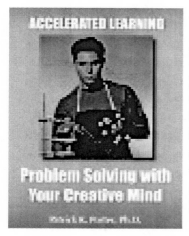

Whether you are an honor student or just having difficulty taking a test, this breakthrough learning system will help you overcome learning challenges and accelerate your current skill level. Imagine doubling your reading speed while improving your memory. Sit back, relax and allow your mind to organize your life, while you build your self-confidence and earn better grades with the our complete learning system.

Setting Goals for Learning Success

Dr. Porter's Pikeville College study proved that the more successful students are those who have an outcome or ultimate goal in mind. With this module you will learn the secrets of goal setting, experience a boost in motivation, and see your self-confidence in the classroom soar.

Being an Optimistic Thinker

Henry Ford once said, "Whether you think you can, or you think you can't, you are right." It all starts with attitude. You will be guided into the creative state, where you'll discover ways of breaking through to your optimistic mind that will help you to think, act and respond with a positive nature even during your most difficult classes or around challenging people.

Six Steps to Using Your Perfect Memory

Harness the natural byproduct of relaxing your mind by using the six steps that activate a perfect memory. You will discover creative ways to access and recall the information you need as you need it! Best of all, you will have this ability the rest of your life.

Check Out The Complete
Accelerated Learning Series
at **www.Self-MasteryTechnology.com**

Dr. Patrick Porter's
Heart Healthy Lifestyle Series
Inspired by the principles of
Dr. Michael Irving's
Twelve Wisdoms to a Healthy Heart

Adversities and life challenges can be viewed as burdens or as gifts. A heart attack or diagnosis of heart disease is a dramatic wakeup call. Dr. Porter and Dr. Irving want you to see your diagnosis as the gift that it is—the opportunity to create a heart-healthy lifestyle and a brand new you!

Download the Demo for Free!
Visit www.12WisdomsToAHealthyHeart.com

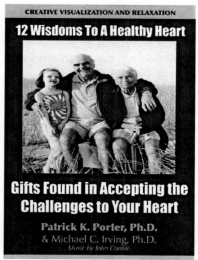

Gifts Found in Accepting the Challenges to Your Heart
A heart crisis can be frightening, but it can also make you feel grateful to be alive and can increase your appreciation of life. These early changes will have you well on your way to living a vibrant life of energy and vitality.

Take Charge with a Strong Heart
Taking charge is one of the most important components of heart health and recovery. Now you can take ownership of your own health and be the central director of your success, confident in your knowledge of heart health, and ready to make the decisions that fulfill your goals.

Check Out The Complete
Heart Healthy Lifestyles Series
at **www.Self-MasteryTechnology.com**

Dr. Patrick Porter's
Freedom From Addiction Series

Addiction comes in many forms, but the underlying cause remains the same. For every addiction there is an underlying positive intention that the mind is trying to fulfill. Now you can use the power of your mind—through creative visualization and relaxation (SMT)—to find more appropriate ways to satisfy that positive intention without the destructive behaviors of the past. Dr. Patrick Porter's groundbreaking SMT program for overcoming addiction can work for just about any addiction including the following:

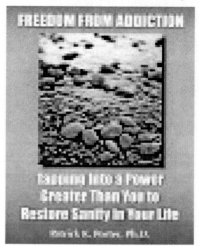

Alcoholism
Anorexia & Bulimia
Codependency
Gambling
Marijuana
Narcotics
Prescription Drugs
Overeating
Overspending
Pornography
Self-Injury
Sexual Promiscuity

Personal Responsibility —Working With Your Other-Than-Conscious Mind to Manage Your Life

Most people who struggle with addictions have, in reality, simply lost their power of choice. Dr. Patrick Porter (PhD) will help you discover why trying to force a change with willpower only perpetuates the problem and how visualization is what will lead you to realization and freedom. You will discover how, by tapping into the power of your mind, you can rebuild your confidence (even in uncertain times) and bring into your consciousness (with sufficient force) the appropriate memories and choices that will lead you to living an addiction-free life—which is your birthright.

Check Out The Complete
Freedom From Addiction Series
at **www.Self-MasteryTechnology.com**

Dr. Patrick Porter's
Coping with Cancer Series

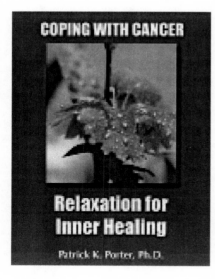

Being diagnosed with cancer is in it-self a stressful event—so stressful it can suppress your immune system and worsen the side-effects of treatment. Fortunately, through guided relaxation, you can let go of your fear and anxiety, and take charge of your recovery. Creative visualization can help you regain an optimistic attitude, spark your immune system, and maximize your medical treatment. If you are ready to join the ranks of people who have discovered the mind/body connection and its healing potential, then the Coping with Cancer Series is definitely for you!

Relaxation For Inner Healing

For some people, relaxing while facing a serious illness may seem like an impossible task. In this first session, you will begin by simply clearing your mind of all negative or fear-based thoughts concerning your condition. At the same time, you will learn to allow the natural healing power of your body to take over. The benefits from relaxation are immeasurable when it comes to fighting cancer.

Rejuvenate Your Body Through Deep Delta Sleep

During cancer recovery, many people have difficulty falling asleep or they may awaken in the middle of the night and struggle to get back to sleep. Your body naturally recharges and rejuvenates during sleep, which means a good night's rest is key to your recovery. This imagery will show you new ways to get maximum benefit from sleep.

Check Out The Complete
Coping With Cancer Series
at **www.Self-MasteryTechnology.com**

Dr. Patrick Porter's
SportZone™ Series

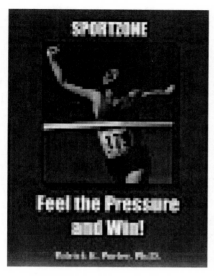

Success in sports is about being the best you can be, and visualization plays a key role in getting there. The SportZone program is designed to help you tap into the mind's potential and make your sport of choice fun and enjoyable while taking your game to the next level. Visualization for sports performance is nothing new to top competitors—athletes from Tiger Woods to diver Greg Louganis and a variety of Olympians have used visualization to bring about optimal performance, overcome self-doubt, and give themselves a seemingly unfair advantage over their competition.

Using the "Zone" in Your Sport

When competitive athletes slip into their "zone" everything seems to work just right. Dr. Patrick Porter will help you get to that place where everything comes together. With this process you'll learn to put yourself into a state of "flow," your own personal "zone," so you can stay on top of your game.

Control Your Emotions and Master Your Sport

It has been said that he or she who angers you conquers you; this is true even if the person who angers you is you! With this process you will learn a powerful self-visualization technique for keeping your emotions under control.

Check Out The Complete
SportZone Series
at **www.Self-MasteryTechnology.com**

Dr. Patrick Porter's
Smoking Cessation Series

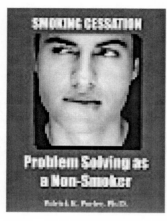

Kicking your smoking habit doesn't get any easier or more fun than this! When you use Dr. Patrick Porter's proven strategies, you'll find that making this life-saving change comes about simply and effortlessly. With the new science of creative visualization and relaxation (SMT), you will extinguish the stress and frustration associated with quitting smoking, and you'll conquer your cravings like the tens of thousands of others who have used Dr. Porter's processes.

Making the Decision To Be A Non-Smoker

With this SMT session, you'll learn about the cleansing power of you own mind, and use it to take a "mental shower" that will wipe away all thoughts of tobacco. With this process, you'll gladly make the decision to be tobacco-free for life!

Making Peace With Your Mind

In this powerful creative session, Dr. Patrick Porter will show you that, while you once had a positive intention for having tobacco in your life, you no longer need it to live the life you desire. The smoker of the past will make peace with the clean air breather of the future in order to create a new, vibrant you!

Plan Your Life As A Non-Smoker

Every goal needs a plan, and in this process, Dr. Patrick Porter will guide you in visualizing and working a plan for your tobacco-free life. This motivational session will allow you to remember to forget cigarettes forever. You'll awake convinced being a nonsmoker is as easy as taking a breath of fresh air!

Check Out The Complete
Smoking Cessation Series
at **www.Self-MasteryTechnology.com**

Dr. Patrick Porter's
Mental Coaching for Golf Series

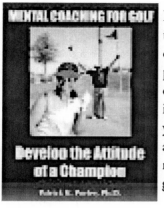

Efficient golfers know how to relax and let their minds take over. Now, thanks to these creative visualization and relaxation (SMT) processes, you'll learn to see yourself as a calm, confident golfer. You deserve to take pleasure in your time on the course. Thanks to SMT, you'll finally be able to let go of frustration and focus on every stroke—meaning you'll not only play better, but you'll also enjoy the game more than ever!

Optimize the Risk Zone for Golf

You've never experienced a practice session like this one! Follow along with Dr. Patrick Porter as he guides you onto the driving range in your mind. Once there, you'll practice each swing, letting go of negative thoughts and allowing the clubs to do what they were designed to do— send the ball straight to the target.

Develop the Attitude of a Champion

Champions understand that good outcomes come from good shots. With this dynamic process, you'll find it easy to think positive thoughts and accept each shot as it comes. You'll no longer spend time feeling distracted, over-analyzing your game, blaming the conditions of the course, or getting angry over a bad lie.

Concentration: Your Key To Consistency

Most golf professionals consider concentration to be the key to playing golf...but almost no one teaches it. In this energizing process by Dr. Patrick Porter, he'll teach you to achieve the concentration you need simply by sitting back, relaxing, and letting go of all stress and confusion.

Check Out The Complete
Mental Coaching for Golf Series
at **www.Self-MasteryTechnology.com**

Dr. Patrick Porter's
Enlightened Children's Series

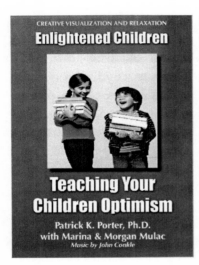

Seven-year-old Marina Mulac and five-year-old Morgan Mulac, who have come to be known as the world's youngest marketers, were the inspiration behind this Enlightened Children's Series. When they met Dr. Patrick Porter, they had one question for him: Why had he created so many great visualizations for grown ups and nothing for kids?

Dr. Porter told the two little entrepreneurs that if they put on their thinking caps and helped him design a program for kids, together they could help children from around the globe to use their imaginative minds to become better people and help improve the world. Together, Marina, Morgan, and Dr. Patrick Porter put together this series that uses guided imagery, storytelling, and positive affirmations to help children see the world as a peaceful and harmonious place where everyone can win. If your goal is to develop a happy, healthy child of influence in our rapidly changing world, this series is a must-have for your child.

Building Optimism in Your Children

Every day your child is forming his or her view of the world based on life experiences. Now is the time to help your child build a positive outlook that will serve him or her for a lifetime. Optimists believe that people and events are inherently good and that most situations work out for the best. Dr. Porter will show your child how to see the good in every situation and how to be open to experiencing new things.

Check Out The Complete
Enlightened Children's Series
at **www.Self-MasteryTechnology.com**

Dr. Patrick Porter's
Medical Series

De-Stress and Lower Blood Pressure

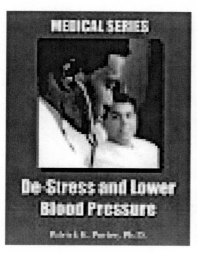

The physiological benefits of deep relaxation and visualization are well documented. During this creative visualization process you will learn to achieve the relaxation response—a state known to unlock your brain's potential for de-stressing your body and returning your blood pressure to a healthy level. Known benefits of the relaxation response also include a lower respiratory rate, a slower pulse, relaxed muscles, and an increase in alpha brain wave activity—everything that makes for a healthier you!

Pre-Surgery Calm for Better Healing

For years physicians and therapist have used guided relaxation, intense concentration, and focused attention to achieve deep relaxation and heightened states of awareness prior to surgery. Now, through the science of Self-mastery Technology (SMT), you can easily benefit from these powerful processes.

Post-Surgery Stress Relief for a
Healthy Mind and Body

SMT is a relaxation technique that uses concentration and deep breathing to calm the mind and put your body in the best possible state for repair and healing. What could be easier than to sit back, relax, and let the stress of surgery and recovery melt away?

Check Out The Complete
Medical Series
at **www.Self-MasteryTechnology.com**

Dr. Patrick Porter's
Professional Airlines Blue Sky Series

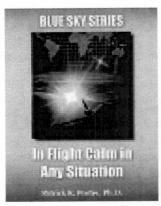

The airline industry has long been considered a "glamour" industry, but those working in the business know that, once it becomes your job, you are in a constant battle to maintain the health of your body and mind. An airline professional's stress can come in many forms—from dealing with exhausting schedules and unruly passengers to the underlying fears related to travel during uncertain times. For this reason, Dr. Patrick Porter, has created the Blue Sky Series, which is designed to help airline professionals regain balance in their lives through deep relaxation and creative visualization techniques.

Sleep on Any Schedule

In the airline industry, flying across time zones, arriving late at night, and being expected to awaken early the next morning are all part of the job. While the occasional traveler is able to get over jet lag with relative ease, in the airline business, jet lag is part and parcel to a day's work. Unfortunately, this regular disruption of the sleep cycle can result in chronic fatigue, headaches, body aches, and a lowered immune system.

Clear Out Flight Noise and Return to Health

With this visualization, you will be guided through some mental balancing processes to help you deal with the impact of that constant barrage of jet engine noise. During the process you will clear your mind, reset your attention, and focus on health. You will learn to de-stress, relax, and have fun after a flight.

Check Out The Complete
Blue Sky Series
at **www.Self-MasteryTechnology.com**

Dr. Patrick Porter's
Pain-Free Lifestyle Series

Persistent pain can have a costly impact on your life. It can lead to depression, loss of appetite, irritability, anger, loss of sleep, withdrawal from social interaction, and an inability to cope. Fortunately, with creative visualization and relaxation (SMT), pain can almost always be controlled. SMT helps you eliminate pain while you relax, revitalize, and rejuvenate. You deserve to be free of your pain—and now you can be, thanks to SMT!

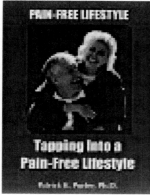

Tapping into a Pain-Free Lifestyle
Dr. Patrick Porter will guide you through a simple exercise to transform pain into relaxation. You'll tap into your body's innate ability to heal itself, allowing the healing process to happen while you take a relaxing mental vacation. Pain will lose all power over you as you learn to relax away your pain and enjoy your life free from discomfort.

Activate Your Mental Pharmacy
In this dynamic process, you'll unlock your body's natural pharmacy, flushing pain from your body and neutralizing all discomfort. You will so galvanize your mind's healing capacity, all you'll have to do is say the word to release pain, fear and anxiety. Most importantly, you'll have this healing power at your fingertips—when and where you need it most.

Starting the Day Pain-Free
In this motivational session, Dr. Patrick Porter will show you that living pain-free is as simple as saying, "So-Hum." Which means, transporting yourself to a pain-free state can be as easy as breathing!

Check Out The Complete
Pain-Free Lifestyle Series
at **www.Self-MasteryTechnology.com**

Dr. Patrick Porter's
Stress-Free Childbirth Series

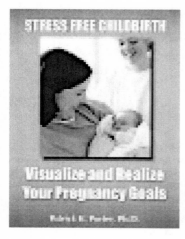

Bringing a child into the world should be an amazing life experience. Sadly, for many women, the joy of the event is lost due to fear, stress and pain. Also, research has shown that a fetus can actually feel the stress, worry, and negative emotions of the mother during pregnancy. This breakthrough series is designed to help the mother-to-be to relax, let go of stress, and enjoy the entire process of pregnancy, delivery and motherhood. In addition, the listener is taught to use the power of thought to create an anaesthetized feeling that can transform pain into pressure throughout labor and delivery—making the entire process stress-free for the entire family.

Visualize and Realize Your Pregnancy Goals

Take this journey of the imagination where you'll train your brain to stay focused and on task. With this process, you'll start experiencing the relaxation response, set healthy priorities, and prepare your body for the many changes it will go through for the next nine months and beyond. This is the foundation session for the complete Stress-Free Childbirth program.

Mental Skills for Pregnancy and Delivery

With this session negative thinking melts away and a calm state of emotional readiness replaces fear. The power of positive expectancy will lead you to positive results. Once you experience this mental training, and gain the relaxed mindset and inner confidence you need for motherhood, others may actually look to you for support!

Check Out The Complete
Stress-Free Childbirth Series
at **www.Self-MasteryTechnology.com**

Dr. Patrick Porter's
Mind-Over-Menopause Series

For many women mid-life can be a time of uncertainty and loss. For some the loss of fertility and the perceived loss of youth can cause depression and anxiety. At the same time, the body's response to the decrease in hormones can create any number of symptoms—hot flash-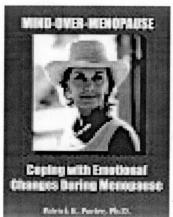es, night sweats, weight gain, itchy skin, mood swings, lost libido, headaches, and irregular cycles are just of few of the meno-pausal challenges women face. Now you can reclaim that woman, along with all the strength, confidence, and wisdom you gained in the first half of your life. This series takes you way beyond mind over matter—it's mind over menopause!

Balance Your Mood, Balance Your Life
With this session you will use creative vi-sualization and relaxation to help balance your mood, harness positive mental energy, and use your innate cre-ative power to produce much-needed balance in your life during this time of change and uncertainty. You will stop focusing on what you've lost, and discover all that you've gained!

Mental Skills to Help You Master Menopause
With this creative visualization and relaxation process, you will be given time to plan your life from a new perspective. You will learn to view menopause as a rite of passage—one that gives you confidence and inner worth. With new ways to handle situations at work, and with family and friends, you'll discover that mid-life can bring forth a whole new you that's been there all along just waiting to blossom!

Check Out The Complete
Mind-Over-Menopause Series
at **www.Self-MasteryTechnology.com**

Dr. Patrick Porter's
Sales Mastery Series

 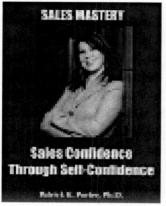

Attend Our Local FREE Weight Loss Seminar

We'd like to invite you to an amazing seminar held right in our office, where you will discover how you can finally lose your weight! You will discover a new breakthrough system that will show you on a day-to-day basis what you can do to get your body into FAT BURNING rather than FAT STORING! You have Fat Burning Hormones that should be working for you! You'll learn what you can do to switch your hormones into Fat Burning mode!

www.clubreduce.com

Learn the Secret to Weight Loss at Club Reduce!

Different weight loss programs are waiting everywhere. When you're having trouble losing weight, it can be nearly impossible to see through the veils and choose the right kind program for you. Although many weight loss programs are initially effective, not many of them offer lasting weight loss or, more importantly, lasting health. At Club Reduce® the objective is to help you lose extra weight, keep that weight off, and feel fantastic!

There are constantly new weight loss programs, fad diets, exercises, and pills coming out as a way to lose weight. A popular craze is the "no fat" craze. This is not effective, because our bodies need unsaturated fats to work properly. When the body isn't working as it should, it holds onto fat as a health precaution and enters a fat storing stage. There are also many weight loss systems that offer (usually their own brand) low calorie snacks or meals. These foods may be low in calories, but are often stuffed full of chemicals, artificial sweeteners or flavors, and other substances that are toxic to consume. The truth is, effective and lasting weight loss will never be found in a plethora of pre-packaged foods, but instead in the wholesome foods the earth provides. Don't fall for a program that doesn't take work on your end, because it takes work to lose weight the healthy way; a decision that is in your own hands.

Club Reduce® is a nationwide collection of natural weight loss clinics started in Salt Lake City, Utah, by Doctor Todd Singleton. There are many different Club Reduce® weight loss programs that all of the clinics use. These programs employ 100% nutrition, detoxification, and all-natural supplements as the foundation for a healthy solution to weight loss. Club Reduce® has aided thousands of people in reaching their weight loss goals, and they can help you too! These programs are designed to help you effectively lose weight while getting the body in ultimate health. The truth is, when the body has everything it needs, unneeded weight will come off without effort. The work is in getting healthy!

There are a lot of ways to learn what Club Reduce® is all about. Two free seminars are offered, one in-office, and one online. You can also register to receive a Free Weight Loss Report that will educate you on some of the basics of healthy and natural weight loss. Though you can schedule to meet for a One-on-One Weight Loss Evaluation without attending these seminars, the seminars will help you better understand what needs to be done to lose weight, and you will receive a Seminar Discount on your Evaluation! Finally drop the weight and feel fantastic! Get your energy and libido back!

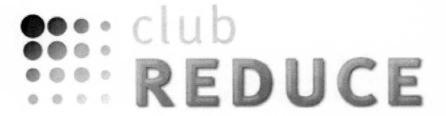

Contact your nearest Club Reduce® Location at:
www.ClubReduce.com

CPSIA information can be obtained at www.ICGtesting.com
Printed in the USA
BVOW04s0825120214

344724BV00001B/8/P